ILLUSTRATED ELEMENTS OF
AROMATHERAPY

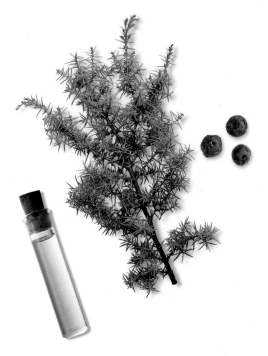

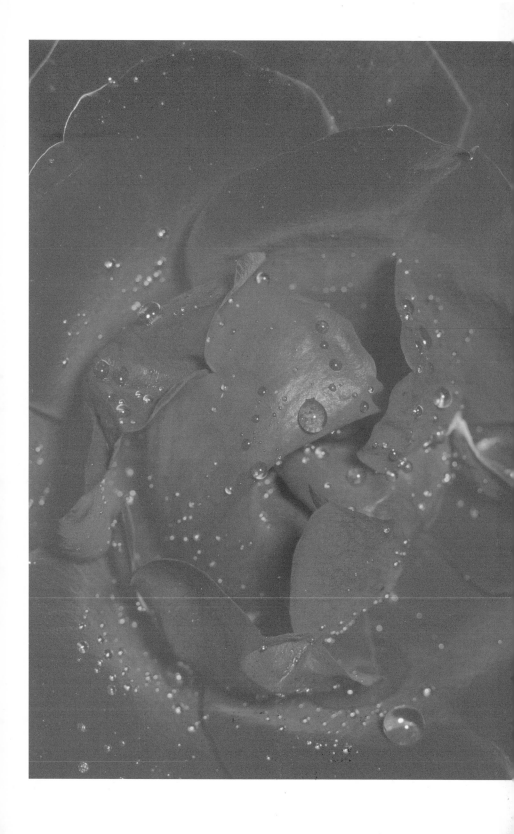

ILLUSTRATED ELEMENTS OF
AROMATHERAPY

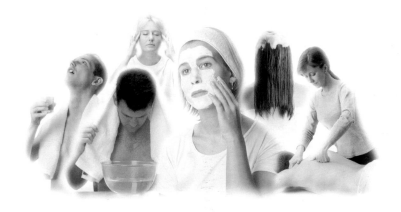

CLARE WALTERS

thorsons

© Element Books Limited 1998
Text © Clare Walters 1998

First published in Great Britain in 1998 by
ELEMENT BOOKS LIMITED
Shaftesbury, Dorset, SP7 9BP

Thorsons
An Imprint of HarperCollins*Publishers*
77-85 Fulham Palace Road
Hammersmith
London W6 8JB

The Thorsons website address is www.thorsons.com

and Thorsons are trademarks of
HarperCollins*Publishers* Limited

First published in Great Britain in 1998 by
ELEMENT BOOKS LIMITED
Shaftesbury, Dorset SP7 9BP

© Text Clare Walters 1998

NOTE FROM THE PUBLISHER
*Any information given in this book is not intended to be taken as a replacement for
medical advice. Any person with
a condition requiring medical attention should consult a qualified practitioner or
therapist.*

Designed and created with
THE BRIDGEWATER BOOK COMPANY LIMITED

Printed and bound in Hong Kong by
Printing Express.

British Library Cataloguing in Publication
data available

Library of Congress Cataloging-in-Publication data available

ISBN 0-00-715046-6

Acknowledgments

*The publisher would like to thank
the following for the use of pictures:*
A–Z Botanical Collection: 24b, 66l, 86l, 108l&b, 118l.
Bridgeman Art Library: 6 (Sotheby's, New York), 10tl
(Bradford Art Galleries and Museums), 11tr (Royal Albert
Memorial Museum, Exeter), 12t (British Museum, London),
14c (Private Collection), 26b (Palazzo della Ragione,
Padua), 49t (Palazzo Ducale, Mantua), 73t (Stapleton
Collection), 75 (Museo Archeologico, Florence), 77t (British
Museum), 85 (Museé des Arts Decoratifs, Paris), 87tr
(British Museum), 103t (Whitford & Hughes, London),
105t (Royal Ontario Museum, Toronto), 107t (V&A,
London), 109 (Private Collection), 115r (Christies Images).
Corbis UK: 107b, 111b.
C. W. Daniel Company: 15tl.
e. t. archive: 10r, 11c, 12b&c, 13t, 14t, 21tl, 55c, 61bl, 63t,
91b, 97t, 99b, 111t.
Garden Picture Library: 20c (J. S. Sira); 48tl, 82l (Marijke
Heuff); 50tl, 60l (Brigitte Thomas); 54tl, 64l, 74l, 90l (Emma
Peios); 56l (Michel Viaro); 58t (Linda Burgess); 62l
(Neil Holmes); 68l (Philippe Bonduel); 70l (Gary Rogers);
76l, 84l (Brian Carter); 78l (Lamontagne); 94l, 100l
(Mayer/Le Scarff); 96l (John Glover); 98l (Jacqui Hurst);
102l (Jerry Pavia); 106l (Michael Viard); 110l (Didier
Willery); 112l (Bob Challinor).
Harry Smith Horticultural Collection: 52l, 104l.
Houses & Interiors Photographic Agency: 80l, 116t.
Hutchison Library: 53r, 117t.
Image Bank: 59t.
NHPA: 92L, 117c.
Robert Harding Picture Library: 95t.
Science Photo Library: 11tl, 65br, 68b, 79, 91br, 139b.
Stock Market: 8, 20l, 29t, 29b, 32, 33, 53l, 65t, 68t, 71r, 72l,
81, 85t, 87tr, 91tr, 93, 97b, 101br, 113, 119.

With thanks to:
William Chaplin, Bonnie Craig, Jessie Fuller, Ray Goldstein,
Nicky Hobby, Julia Holden, Simon Holden,
Helen Irvine, Kevin Irvine, Helen Jordan,
Chloe Knight, Pat Knight, Jane Manze,
Andrew Milne, Kay Macmullan, Jan Phillips,
Sam Sains, Amelia Whitelaw, Gabriel Whitelaw
for help with photography

Special thanks to:
The Plinth Company, Stowmarket, Suffolk

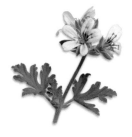

Contents

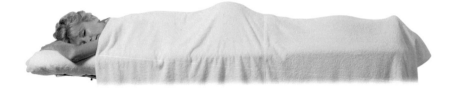

Preface

AROMATHERAPY HAS *been around in some form or another for thousands of years, and our sense of smell is integral to how we perceive the world. In this book I hope to show what a delight essential oils are, and how easily and effectively they can be used. An understanding of aromatherapy will allow you to fill your home with aromas that are both beautiful and therapeutic. You can also use aromatherapy to alleviate a wide variety of stress-related conditions. In these situations the combination of powerful essential oils and the therapeutic, loving touch of a massage can be incredibly potent.*

ABOVE *This incense burner was used in 18th century China.*

The only thing I would emphasize to anyone using oils for the first time is that they contain pure, concentrated plant energy and must be treated with respect. It takes thousands of petals to make just one drop of rose or jasmine oil, for example. All essential oils are strong and you must take care when using them. This book contains cautions and contraindications, and it is important that you read them and take them to heart.

Practising aromatherapists will find enough detail on the 36 oils included in the Materia Medica, as well as general information elsewhere, to enjoy this book as a reference guide. I hope the oils give you as much pleasure as they have already given me. Each one has its own individual characteristics and idiosyncrasies, and if you use them regularly you may well come to regard them as trusted friends.

BELOW *Oils contain pure plant energy and must be used with care.*

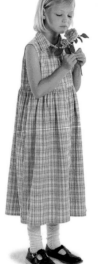

LEFT *Young and old alike can enjoy the scent of a beautiful flower.*

How to use this book

The first part of the book provides an introduction to the art of aromatherapy and its history. Aromatherapy oils, their preparation, and chemical make-up, and the ways in which they can be blended, stored, and used are then covered. A detailed section on massage follows. The extensive Materia Medica is a thorough reference guide to the principal oils. The final part of the book explains the ways in which the oils can be used in the home, ending with a glossary, bibliography, and list of useful addresses, as well as a comprehensive index.

Each new topic is introduced with an opening paragraph that provides a clear outline of the subject.

BELOW **As well as discussing the history of aromatherapy, its origins and efficacy, the first part of the book also explains how to use the oils to make your own lotions and potions at home.**

Techniques are described and shown visually, using step-by-step photography.

BELOW **Massage is a fundamental technique in aromatherapy. Clear photographic step-by-step sequences explain the different massage strokes that can be used with the essential oils.**

BELOW **Aromatherapy has a host of benefits for all the family, and especially for women and children. These are highlighted in a special section after the Materia Medica reference guide.**

Wherever necessary, advice is given on how to improve your technique and how to avoid problems.

Practical hints and tips are provided throughout the book.

Clear photographs show precisely what to do in order to gain the greatest benefits from aromatherapy.

Combinations of oils are recommended for particular physical ailments and conditions.

What is Aromatherapy?

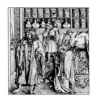

ABOVE *The healing value of plants has been recognized by herbalists for centuries.*

AROMATHERAPY IS *the use of therapeutic oils extracted from natural plant matter in order to encourage good health, equilibrium, and well-being. The essential oils that are used in aromatherapy are truly holistic in that they can have a powerful and positive effect on mind, body, and spirit. To use the essential oils well it is necessary to take time to understand a little of the essence of the person you are choosing them for, whether you are using the oils for yourself or another.*

Essential oils are extracted from trees, bushes, flowers, and shrubs from all over the world and each oil has its own unique chemical make-up. In the last 40 years research has brought together plants from all five continents into a form that is now both a science and an art. The origins of aromatherapy seem to go back as far as the origins of man, though the term aromatherapy is itself fairly new. The scientific study of the essential oils is both replacing and validating the instinctive and trusting responses of indigenous peoples and traditional folklore. Many oils from the far-flung corners of the world have been respected for their therapeutic effects for many years, and now these effects are being studied scientifically. Research into the oils is ongoing, and in many cases discoveries are validating what has seemingly always been traditionally accepted in folklore.

The principal healing chemicals of many essential oils have more

BELOW *Each oil has a different chemical make-up according to its plant source.*

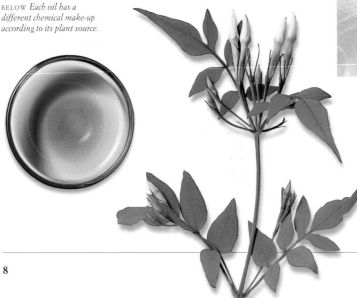

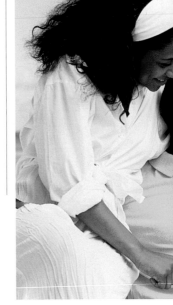

ABOVE *The use of essential oils will benefit the whole family and contribute to a stress-free life.*

LEFT *This jasmine plant is one of many plants from around the world used to produce essential oils.*

recently been extracted for use in allopathic medicine, but it is the many trace elements that give each oil its essential quality and its unique ability to heal. Essential oils are rich, organic compounds with a complex chemical structure.

One of the main contemporary uses of essential oils is to alleviate the various symptoms of chronic stress ranging from insomnia to dyspepsia to migraines. This, however, is by no means the only condition that aromatherapy can alleviate.

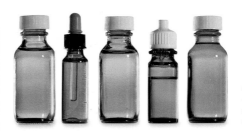

LEFT *Store your essential oils properly and keep them out of the reach of children.*

The magic of the oils is that they can affect the whole person: their physical symptoms, attitude, and mood. Refer to "Aromatherapy in the Home" (*see pp. 120–135*) for a list of common ailments, experienced by both adults and children, and the various oils with which they can be treated.

Keep the bottles out of reach of children and do not take the oils internally unless they are prescribed for you by a properly qualified physician or other practitioner. Be careful also, when you are using the oils at home to keep them out of your eyes and mouth. Take particular care to thoroughly wash your hands after working with the oils, especially if you are using neat oil and resist any temptation you have to try adding them to food and

drink like the edible plants they come from. Essential oils are far more concentrated than any preparation you might buy for food use. Particular cautions for use and any circumstances in which an oil should be avoided completely are indicated in the Materia Medica.

As long as you are careful you need never worry about using any essential oils. They are natural energies and if you respect the power of the concentrated healing and nurturing energy you are working with, the oils will both give you great pleasure and lend their therapeutic gifts to help you deal with many ailments, conditions, and challenges in your life. There are far more advantages than disadvantages to using the oils.

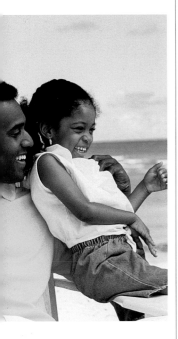

CAUTION

Always consult your physician if you are worried about any medical condition.

MAKE TIME FOR YOURSELF

Whether you use the oils at home or visit a professional therapist, taking time for yourself can be very beneficial. You may choose to treat yourself to a relaxing massage, benefiting from both the touch of the person giving you the massage and the oils chosen for your healing. Or you can simply add the oils to the bath, or use them in a vaporizer, to calm your thoughts and aid restful sleep.

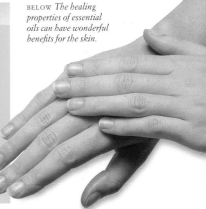

BELOW *The healing properties of essential oils can have wonderful benefits for the skin.*

The Origins of Aromatherapy

THE HEALING *power of plants has been acknowledged by many cultures for thousands of years, and aromatherapy can be said to stem from the various systems of traditional medicine developed by ancient civilizations. Primitive peoples used plants in both their healing traditions as well as in their religious rituals. As an example, pollen traces of therapeutic plants have been found by archeologists in burial sites and dwellings of primitive humans.*

ABOVE *Incense has traditionally been used in the church or temple as a spiritual tool.*

Plants are the most natural and easily obtainable form of nourishment and our ancestors must have noticed that edible roots, berries, or leaves of certain plants had a physical effect over and above that of starving off hunger pangs, or that certain extracted plant juices helped wounds to heal faster. They would also have noticed which plants the animals ate and the effects of these plants. Knowledge of this kind was considered precious and was handed down within a tribe from one generation to the next.

Primitive people recognized that smoke, created by burning different woods, also had a variety of effects – perhaps the tribal people became drowsy, or happy, or maudlin; or perhaps someone had a spiritual experience.

LEFT *Plant lore developed over the centuries as our ancestors noticed the physical effects of various berries, roots, and leaves.*

The process of "smoking the sick" (wafting aromatic smoke over patients) subsequently developed into one of the earliest forms of healing. In some parts of the world aromatic smoke continues to be used for its healing powers, indeed it was used in French hospitals until relatively recently. Modern scientific research has verified the antiseptic and bactericidal properties of many of the woods traditionally used. Special or magical smoke also inspired (literally) the origins of early religious beliefs and incense is still used today as a spiritual and meditative tool.

The idea of a relationship between humankind and a divinity or spirit was one of the earliest forms of human thought. All indigenous cultures also share a common acceptance of the belief that the growth and continued existence of humanity is dependent on a healthy relationship between the body and

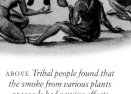

ABOVE *Tribal people found that the smoke from various plants or woods had varying effects on their mood or health.*

the mind and between the gods and humankind. When a person falls ill it reflects a state of disharmony between that person, their environment, and the spirit world, however that world may be envisioned. Consequently the earliest acts of healing endeavored to appease the gods or spirits, as well as to heal the body. In many cultures, fragrant odors were thought to please the gods and healing herbs were even thought to have magical qualities.

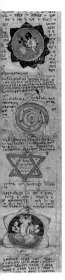

ABOVE
This Sanskrit manuscript instructs Ayurvedic physicians in the use of herbal remedies.

INDIA

Indian medicine is traditionally plant-based. The most ancient of Indian religious writings contain prescriptions and formulae, as well as invocations and prayers, that address the healing plants themselves. Ashoka, a 3rd-century B.C.E. Buddhist king, organized and itemized the cultivation of many medicinal plants that are still used today. The medicinal plants of India became famous throughout Asia, and many have now found their way into Western medical treatments and aromatherapy. India's age-old Ayurvedic medical system is increasingly popular in the West as more people become disillusioned with chemical preparations and turn instead to traditional and holistic forms of healing.

BELOW *These are some of the plants that have been traditionally used in India, China, and Egypt since ancient times.*

CHINA

Traditional Chinese medicine is an ancient system of healing that has survived into the present. Herbal medicine is used in conjunction with acupuncture; the insertion of fine needles into specific points of the body to free its energies. Many Chinese herbs have been used for thousands of years. The earliest known medicinal records in China are in the *Yellow Emperor's Book of Internal Medicine,* which dates from 2000 B.C.E. The great classic of Chinese herbal medicine, known as *Pen ts'ao kang-mou,* lists over 8,000 formulae, most of them plant-based – a greater range of plants than has ever been used in any other system of medicine.

BELOW *The Chinese have a herbal tradition that dates back thousands of years.*

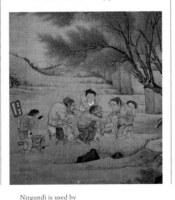

EGYPT

Essential oils have been used in Egypt since the time of the pharaohs. There are records on clay tablets of cedarwood and cypress being imported into Egypt, so even in ancient times there was an international trade in essential oils. By 3500 B.C.E. the priestesses in Egyptian temples were burning gums and resins such as frankincense to clear the mind and as agents in the mummification process. Cedarwood and myrrh were both used very effectively in the embalming process; biochemical research has now shown that cedarwood oil contains a strong fixative, and that myrrh is an excellent antiseptic and antibacterial oil. The oils were also used in other spheres of life – Cleopatra, for example, is said to have harnessed the power of rose oil in order to blind Mark Antony with her charms. Egyptian high priests recorded what they knew about the oils on papyrus and their knowledge forms part of the basis of modern aromatherapy.

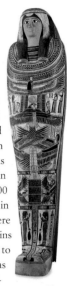

ABOVE *The Egyptians used aromatic oils, such as myrrh and cedar, in embalming.*

Fenugreek is an important medicine in India.

Nirgundi is used by Ayurvedic physicians in their medicines.

Ginger has been used in Chinese medicine for centuries.

Myrrh is native to north-east Africa and was used by the Ancient Egyptians.

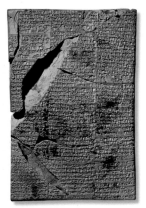

ABOVE *Tablets from Babylon
record the preparations used
by the physicians in their
remedies and treatments.*

BABYLON

Babylonian doctors recorded their prescriptions on clay tablets but, unlike the Egyptians, they did not record what quantities to use. Presumably this was general knowledge. What they did record was what time of day the preparations should be prepared and used – usually at sunrise.

GREECE

The ancient Greeks gained much of their knowledge of essential oils from the Egyptians, but they also acknowledged that the aroma of certain flowers could be either uplifting or relaxing. They used olive oil in their enfleurage processes. The Greek physician Hippocrates (c. 469–399 B.C.E.), who was revered as the father of medicine, refers to a vast number of medicinal plants in his writings.

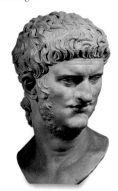

ABOVE *The Emperor Nero
used rose oil as a remedy
for headaches.*

ROME

Many Greek physicians were employed by the Romans, and through them the use of medicinal plants gradually spread around the ancient world. The Romans used essential oils for pleasure – to perfume their hair, bodies, and clothes – as well as for pain relief. They also used oils in massage, especially after bathing. Rose oil was the Emperor Nero's favorite: it cured his headaches and relieved his indigestion. The Romans also used chamomile to treat skin complaints and to help in the healing of wounds. It is now known to contain azulene, which is a natural anti-inflammatory agent.

After the fall of Rome many physicians fled to Constantinople, taking their knowledge with them. Here the works of the great Graeco-Roman physicians, such as Galen and Hippocrates, were painstakingly translated into Arabic and their knowledge spread throughout the Arab world.

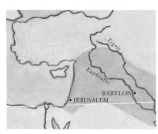

ABOVE *Essential oils were
used by physicians in the
kingdom of Babylonia,
situated between the Tigris
and Euphrates rivers.*

RIGHT *The works
of the great Graeco-
Roman physicians were
translated into Arabic.*

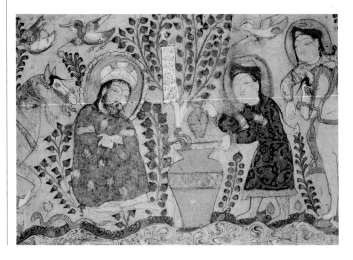

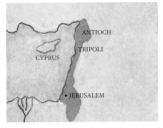

ABOVE *The use of herbal oils spread to Europe from the Middle East in the 11th and 12th centuries.*

EUROPE

What happened in Europe during the Dark Ages, after the fall of Rome, is unclear, although the widespread persecution of "witches" for their "magical" healing powers indicates that there must have been a strong folk healing tradition at that time, one that would have included the use of aromatic plants.

By the 12th century the concept of aromatherapy had definitely arrived in Europe. During the Crusades, European barber surgeons worked alongside Arab physicians, learning from them the importance of hygiene and the uses of oils. Knights returning from the Crusades brought the herbs and oils back to Europe, along with an understanding of the steam-distillation process. European perfumers, such as the famous French perfume house at Grasse, then began to experiment with local plants.

The invention of the printing press in the 15th century led to the rapid spread of knowledge, and recipes and methods were frequently gathered together and published as "herbals." During this time floors were often strewn with

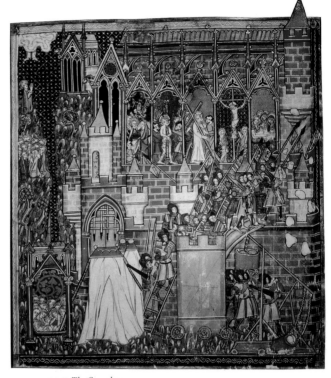

ABOVE *The Crusaders learned about oils while fighting in the East.*

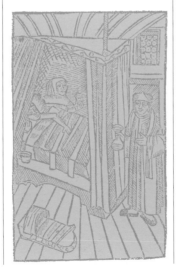

herbs that gave off their volatile oils when walked on, and little bouquets of herbs, known as "tussie-mussies," were carried in public places to ward off infection. In 1665, the year of the Great Plague in Britain, people in London burned lavender, cedarwood, and cypress in the streets. These practices have often been dismissed by historians as little more than superstition, but many of the preparations that were used are now known to be disinfectants, bactericides, and antiviral agents, or insecticides and insect repellents.

LEFT *Protective bouquets of herbs were placed in the sick room as an aid against the Plague during the 17th Century.*

Aromatherapy Through the Ages

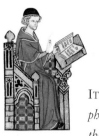

ABOVE *Avicenna left valuable records of the plants he used in healing.*

IT WAS NOT UNTIL *1928 that the term aromatherapie was coined by a French pharmacist but the growth of aromatherapy as we know it can be traced from the works of Avicenna in Arabia to the present day. Folklore and medical practice have gradually converged to give us a science that resides in respecting the healing properties of the essence of naturally grown plant matter.*

AVICENNA *980–1037*

The greatest Arab physician of early times was Abu Ali Ibn Sina, known in the West as Avicenna. He was physician-in-chief to the hospital in Baghdad and personal physician to a succession of caliphs. Avicenna described more than 800 medicinal species of plant, but it is not possible to identify them all since he used their Indian, Tibetan, and Chinese vernacular names. They included lavender, chamomile, and rose.

Avicenna invented traction for broken limbs and used manipulation for structural abnormalities. He also wrote instructions on massage, including techniques for sports massage that would be acceptable today. His importance for aromatherapy is his discovery of the steam-distillation process. Arab manuscripts have drawings of distillation equipment that, albeit less sophisticated than that used today, differs little in its basic principle.

Avicenna was also an alchemist, placing great significance on red and white roses in his experiments, and attar of roses was produced in Persia during his lifetime.

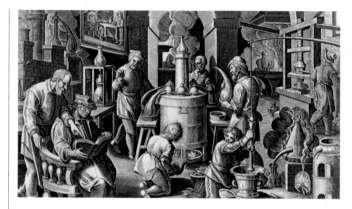

NICHOLAS CULPEPER *1616–1654*

The astrologer and physician Nicholas Culpeper incurred the wrath of the Royal College of Physicians by translating the *Pharmacopoeia* from Latin into

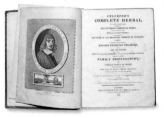

ABOVE *Culpeper's Complete Herbal was first published in 1653.*

ABOVE *This 16th century engraving shows the distillation of herbs.*

English. This meant that the information contained in it was no longer the exclusive property of physicians, and other Latin scholars. The book, known generally as "Culpeper's herbal," gave clear descriptions of medicinal plants and the places they could be found. Culpeper intended the book to be used by ordinary people. He gave precise information on how to prepare the plant material, and suggested that infused herbs should be used to anoint, or massage, an afflicted person.

RENÉ GATTEFOSSÉ
1881–1950

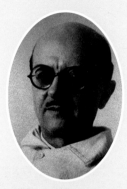

It was in 1928 that the French chemist René Gattefossé coined the term *aromatherapie*. His research work was the result of an accident suffered while working in the laboratory of a perfumery. He badly burned his hand and plunged it into the nearest bowl of liquid, which happened to be neat lavender oil. The hand healed very quickly and with virtually no scarring. Gattefossé realized that the healing properties of the lavender oil were much greater than those of the synthetic preparations that he had been working on. He then began researching the healing properties of other essential oils, taking into consideration their chemical properties as well as their smells.

BELOW *Gattefossé discovered that lavender has great healing properties, and is one of the few oils that can be safely used neat on the skin.*

AROMATHERAPY TODAY

In France aromatherapists are exclusively either physicians or beauty therapists. However, in the rest of Europe, the U.S., Australia, and Canada a strand of aromatherapy has developed that is based on a holistic approach, seeking to treat the body as a whole and promote health on all levels. These aromatherapists choose oils that work on several levels: mental, physical, and psychological. Essential oils lend themselves to a sensitive and subtle approach, for each one has many properties – unlike either synthetic drugs or the isolated parts of a plant often used in allopathic medicine. Essential oils are frequently balancing in their effect, able, for example, to help the body return from the imbalanced state that caused an illness to a state of ideal balance that represents health and well-being. The same principle of balance applies on the mental and emotional planes. An experienced professional aromatherapist can look beyond the physical application of the oils to help the whole person balance mind, body, and spirit to attain holistic health.

BELOW *Massage is an ideal therapy in the holistic treatment of the body.*

MARGUERITE MAURY
1895–1968

Marguerite Maury, a French bio-chemist, became interested in aromatherapy in the World War II period, using it in combination with other natural health remedies and beauty products. She developed a separate strand of aromatherapy in France, that employed the oils externally, rather than internally, and combined them with massage.

JEAN VALNET
Contemporary

This French physician added to Gattefossé's research while working as a surgeon in World War II. Medical supplies were short and Dr. Valnet found that essential oils frequently proved a very effective substitute. The work of Valnet, Gattefossé, and several other researchers greatly helped to further the scientific validation of aromatherapy, especially as part of the French medical tradition.

15

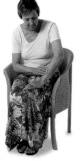

How Aromatherapy Works

ESSENTIAL OILS *enter the body in several different ways. They are absorbed through the skin, passing into the circulatory system. They can also be inhaled, passing into the blood stream through the lungs or, by causing signals to be transmitted through the nervous system directly into the limbic system of the brain.*

ABOVE *Oils can enter the body through the skin.*

Molecules of smell dissolve in the nasal mucus, which is produced by the outer tissue in the nose (olfactory epithelium). This tissue has an area of less than 1sq. in. (6sq. cm.) but is packed with millions of receptors. Each chemoreceptor cell has two extensions: one that leads to the surface of the skin on the inside of the nose and one that reaches back to connect with the nerve fibers at the base of the epithelium. Nerve impulses travel along the fibers through the ethmoid bone in the roof of the mouth and into the cranial cavity. Here, the nerve fibers combine to form the olfactory bulbs and pathways that lead directly back into the limbic system.

The limbic system was one of the earliest parts of the human brain to develop in evolutionary terms. It is where our memories, instincts, and vital functions are controlled. This is why an aroma can be so evocative and so fundamental, whether it is the aroma of fresh bread, coffee, roses, or disinfectant. Every other

sensory experience – even touch – has much further to travel through the nervous system before it is registered, and that registration takes place in a more sophisticated part of the brain. The sense of smell is a very basic instinct. The limbic system registers the existence of a specific oil molecule, and in response the brain releases chemicals that communicate with the

nervous system to relax or stimulate it. These chemicals can also affect the body physically, which is why essential oils can be so effective in the relief of pain.

RIGHT *Aromas enter the limbic system of the brain via the nasal cavity.*

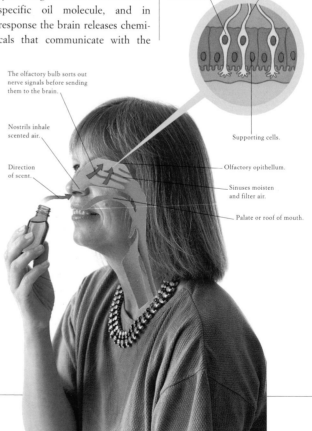

The nose contains 10 million of these receptor cells.

Nerves send signals to olfactory lobe.

The olfactory bulb sorts out nerve signals before sending them to the brain.

Nostrils inhale scented air.

Direction of scent.

Supporting cells.

Olfactory opithellum.

Sinuses moisten and filter air.

Palate or roof of mouth.

A very small quantity of essential oil molecules can, as air is inhaled, become part of the gaseous-exchange between the alveoli, or small air sacs, of the lungs and the thin-walled capillaries. Incoming oxygen is exchanged for outgoing carbon dioxide and the therapeutic essential oil molecules can pass into the body's circulatory system at the same time.

If you put oils on the skin during a massage in a cream or lotion, or in the bath water, they can act on the epidermis (outer layer of the skin) locally. The molecules in the oil are extremely small and can pass through the epidermis to the dermis; the layer of the skin that gives it its pliability. As the dermis is well supplied with capillaries, the oil molecules can pass from the dermis into the capillaries and into the rest of the circulatory system.

Unlike chemical drugs, essential oils do not appear to remain in the body's systems. They are expelled from the body in a variety of ways – through urine, feces, sweat, and exhalation. In a healthy body essential oils remain for no longer than 3–6 hours, and in an unhealthy body they are expelled after approximately 14 hours. The methods of bodily excretion differ according to the particular essential oil used in the preparation. For example, the aromas of sandalwood and juniper oils can be detected in urine, while geranium oil is eliminated in perspiration.

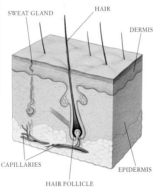

SWEAT GLAND   HAIR

DERMIS

CAPILLARIES

HAIR FOLLICLE   EPIDERMIS

RIGHT *Oil molecules can easily enter the circulatory system through the layers of the skin.*

THE CIRCULATORY SYSTEM

The circulatory system is the main transport system of the body. Essential oils are absorbed into the body's circulatory system via the skin or the mucosa. Once in the bloodstream the oil molecules can travel through it to the areas where they are most needed or can do most good.

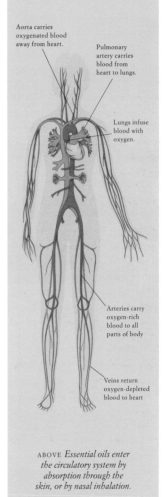

Aorta carries oxygenated blood away from heart.

Pulmonary artery carries blood from heart to lungs.

Lungs infuse blood with oxygen.

Arteries carry oxygen-rich blood to all parts of body

Veins return oxygen-depleted blood to heart

ABOVE *Essential oils enter the circulatory system by absorption through the skin, or by nasal inhalation.*

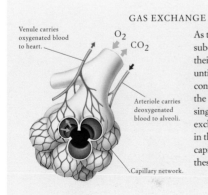

GAS EXCHANGE

Venule carries oxygenated blood to heart.

O_2 CO_2

Arteriole carries deoxygenated blood to alveoli.

Capillary network.

As the air passages in the lungs subdivide to become smaller, their walls become thinner until the muscles and connective tissue that make up the cell walls are replaced by a single layer of cells. The exchange of gases between air in the alveoli and blood in the capillaries takes place across these two fine membranes.

How to Use Essential Oils

ESSENTIAL OILS *are extremely easy and safe to use at home. They may be used simply for their wonderful aromas or you may wish to use them for their cosmetic and medicinal qualities. Whatever your reason, there are many ways in which you can experience the benefits of their soothing and healing properties. Experiment with the different ways that you can use essential oils until you find the method that suits you best.*

ABOVE *Add a few drops of your favorite oil to your bathwater for a sensuous and relaxing experience.*

COMPRESSES

For hot compresses, add a few drops of oil to a bowl of very hot water. Soak a clean cloth or bandage in the water. Wring out the excess, and place the cloth over the area of the body that is affected. Repeat as often as is necessary. Cold compresses can be made in a similar way, using cold water or even ice.

OINTMENTS

Ointments can be made by adding essential oils to a cream base. Refer to "Homemade Preparations" (*pp. 30–31*) for instructions on making your own creams. Alternatively, add your own oils to commercially produced plain, unscented creams.

USE IN THE BATH

Adding oils to a hot bath allows them to come into contact with the whole of the skin at the same time as they are being inhaled into the respiratory system. Four to six drops is all that is needed to fill the room with scented steam. If you use neat oils in the bath, it is extremely important to break up the oil on the surface of the water to avoid the oil burning your skin. The top of the

HOW TO DO A PATCH TEST

If you are trying an oil at home for the first time, whether it is an essential oil or a carrier, always do a patch test before using it on the skin. This is particularly important if you have sensitive skin, suffer from skin allergies, or want to use the oil on a child. Put a drop of the oil on a cotton bud and apply it to the crease of your elbow, the back of your wrist, or under your arm. Put a band-aid over the patch to keep out any water and leave for 24 hours. If there is an adverse reaction to the oil in the form of itching or redness, do not continue to use the oil.

BELOW *The ways in which you can use essential oils are many and varied.*

milk or a drop of vodka can be added to the bath to spread the oil evenly. Alternatively, mix yourself a bottle of bath oil using 3tbsp. (45ml.) of carrier oil, 1tsp. (5ml.) of wheatgerm oil, and 15–20 drops of essential oil. Shake well before use, then add approximately 1tsp. (5ml.) of the oil each time you have a bath.

USE IN MASSAGE

During an aromatherapy massage, the aromatic molecules of the essential oil have a therapeutic effect both through inhalation and through absorption into the skin. The absorption process continues long after the massage has ended.

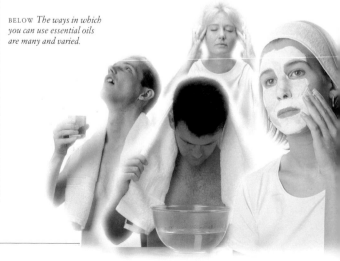

STEAM INHALATIONS

Steam inhalation helps to clear the lungs and sinuses of congestion and infection. Add two or three drops of essential oils to a bowl of steaming hot water. Place your face over the bowl, drape a towel over your head, and breathe in the steam for a few minutes. Rest for a while and then repeat. Discontinue if you feel any discomfort, although you should find that your head clears in a very short time. This method directly affects the respiratory tract and the blood supply.

DIRECT APPLICATION

There are a few specific occasions in first aid when applying neat essential oil directly to a trouble spot is safe. Inhaling the oil straight from the bottle or from a handkerchief can also be helpful, although inhaling too many types of oil in one go – for example, when you are trying to choose which oil to buy – can bring on a headache. Refer to "Aromatherapy in the Home" (see pp. 120–31) for individual conditions and how best to treat them with essential oils.

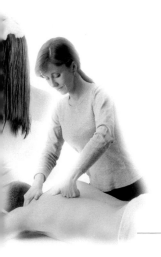

METHODS OF VAPORIZATION

There is a wide variety of equipment available on the market that allows you to perfume your environment and gently release the oils into the atmosphere. These vaporizers can be attractive and fun, especially if you want to share the beauty of the oils with others.

BURNERS
There are many attractive burners available on the market. To use a burner, fill the bowl with water, add one or two drops of oil, and light the candle. Electrical burners have an electric element instead of a nightlight.

SAUCERS
Simply fill a saucer or small bowl with very hot water and add one or two drops of oil.

AROMASTONES
The aromastone plugs into the wall socket. Oil is poured directly onto its heated surface (no water is needed).

LIGHTBULB RINGS
Lightbulb rings sit on top of lightbulbs. When it is turned on the heat of the bulb causes the oils to vaporize.

RADIATOR DIFFUSERS
These fit onto radiators, the heat from the radiator causing the oil to vaporize in the same way as a lightbulb ring.

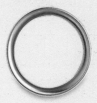

LIGHTBULB RING

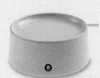

BURNERS   RADIATOR DIFFUSER   AROMASTONE

ABOVE Use whichever method of vaporization you prefer to scent you home.

CAUTION
Never leave a lit candle unattended. • Always ensure a burner or saucer is placed on a heatproof surface. • Never apply essential oils directly to a lightbulb.

CAUTION
Essential oils should never be taken internally, unless prescribed and administered by a medically qualified practitioner. • When using neat oils in the bath, break up the oil on the water's surface with the top of the milk or a drop of vodka to avoid the oil burning your skin.

Preparation of Essential Oils

STEAM DISTILLATION *is the only process that produces a true essential oil. The other oils on the market today are produced by a variety of methods, and contain substances other than the pure essential oil itself. Essential oils are often standardized for use in the food and perfume industries, and consequently are not 100 percent "essential." Aromatherapy forms only a very small part of this vast industry.*

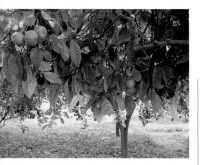

ABOVE *An orchard of oil-yielding citrus fruits.*

There can be a wide variation of quality in the oils available and some manufacturers set higher standards than others. Where the oil crop is grown, under what conditions and with what fertilizers, are important factors in determining the quality and uniqueness of an oil.

STEAM DISTILLATION

This is the most common method of production. When the plant material is heated during the distillation process, only very tiny molecules evaporate, and it is these molecules that make up a true essential oil.

CARBON DIOXIDE EXTRACTION

This technique uses carbon dioxide to explode the molecules of the plant and release the oil. The oils produced are both pure and stable, however, the apparatus for this process is both vast and expensive.

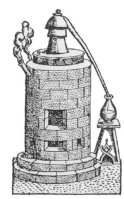

ABOVE *This 16th century engraving shows the way in which plants were distilled.*

BELOW *Steam distillation is the best method of extracting a pure essential oil.*

THE NOTES OF AN OIL

The volatile quality of an oil, or the rate at which it vaporizes, may be described in the same terms as a musical chord. High "notes" have the smallest molecules and the highest volatility, then come the middle notes, and lastly the so-called base notes, with the heaviest and least volatile molecules.

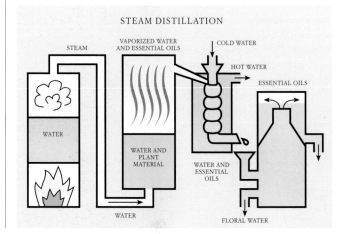

STEAM DISTILLATION

STEAM — VAPORIZED WATER AND ESSENTIAL OILS — COLD WATER — HOT WATER — ESSENTIAL OILS — WATER — WATER AND PLANT MATERIAL — WATER AND ESSENTIAL OILS — WATER — FLORAL WATER

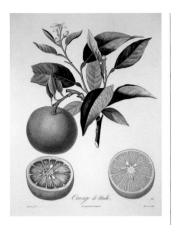

RESINOIDS

A resin is a substance that issues from the bark of a wounded tree and hardens to a solid or semisolid state on exposure to the air. Various solvents are used to extract the aromatic particles from the resin. The solvents are then removed to create pure resins (if an alcohol is used) or resinoids (if a hydrocarbon solvent is used).

LEFT *Citrus oils are extracted by simple expression or pressure.*

CONCRETES

The main difference between a resinoid and a concrete is that various types of plant material (bark, flowers, leaves, herbs, and roots, instead of resin) are used and a solvent is employed to extract the aromatic material. This is the process that is used to produce jasmine oil.

EXPRESSION

This is the method of extraction used for citrus fruits. The oil is squeezed from sacs in the peel and rind of the fruit. The fruit peel can be steam-distilled after expression but this produces oil of an inferior quality. Oils produced by expression have a shorter life than steam-distilled oils. Note that these oils can also cloud with wax if kept in cold conditions; the wax is harmless and can be strained off.

BELOW *Oil is extracted from the Scots pine tree by steam distillation from its needles, cones, and twigs.*

ABSOLUTES

An absolute is created out of a concrete by adding an alcohol to extract the aromatic particles of oil. Frequently some alcohol remains.

SOLVENT EXTRACTION

Resinoids, concretes, and absolutes are highly concentrated perfume materials that contain whatever plant molecules are able to dissolve in the solvent used to extract them. The solvent, however, can never be completely removed from the resultant oil.

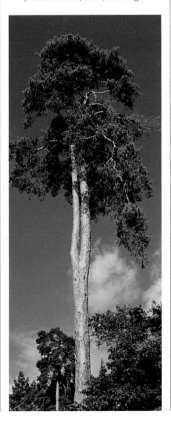

ENFLEURAGE

A pomade is traditionally made by spreading petals or leaves on a tray of animal fat and leaving them until the smell has been absorbed by the fat. The process is then repeated until the fat smells strong enough. It is then treated with alcohol to remove the fat and leave the plant oil. This technique has largely been replaced by the production of concretes.

BELOW *Sandalwood oil is made by water or steam distillation from the dried and powdered roots and heartwood.*

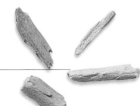

The Chemical Components of Essential Oils

THE CHEMISTRY *of living things is called organic chemistry, or the chemistry of the carbon compound, since all living things contain carbon. In chemical terms, the elements carbon, nitrogen, hydrogen, and oxygen are the units of life.*

ABOVE *Every living thing contains carbon.*

Each of these elements is made up of atoms, once believed to be the smallest particles existent in the universe. When atoms join together they form molecules, and an iso-prene unit is a molecule that is made up of five carbon atoms. Essential oils are mainly based on an isoprene framework, the differences between them resulting from the differences in the types of atoms that attach themselves to the frame-work and the ways in which they are attached. The compounds in essen-tial oils can be separated into dis-tinct chemical groups, each with different properties.

In the descriptions of individual oils in the Materia Medica (*see pp. 46–119*), reference is made to some of the main components, or chemi-cal constituents of each oil. A very basic knowledge of the properties and makeup of an essential oil's components will give you a better understanding of what it does and how it works.

RIGHT *Menthol, which has a cooling aroma, is derived from a terpene.*

TERPENES

Terpenes are made up of varying numbers of isoprene units, and include monoterpenes, sesquiter-penes, and diterpenes. They are generally quite weak in their effect, but they have secondary uses that complement the more powerful components of the oil.

Monoterpenes

Two isoprene units joined together make a monoterpene. They are anti-septic, bactericidal, stimulating, expectorant, and slightly analgesic, although their effects are slight. Some are antiviral and others can break down gallstones. Although used in aromatherapy, they can be skin irritants.

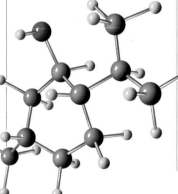

Sesquiterpenes

A vast number of essential oils contain sesquiterpenes, which are made up of three isoprene units. Sesquiterpenes can be antiseptic, bactericidal, hypotensive, calming, and anti-inflammatory, and some can be analgesic or spasmolytic. Scientific researchers have taken a great interest in sesquiterpenes recently as they have been found contain significant anti-inflamma-tory and bactericidal properties.

Diterpenes

Diterpenes are made up of four iso-prene units and rarely make it through the steam-distillation process as they are very heavy in molecular terms. Their action is slightly bactericidal, expectorant, and purgative. Some diterpenes have antifungal and antiviral prop-erties, and may have a positive effect on the endocrine system.

ALCOHOLS

Members of this group are formed when units consisting of one hydro-gen atom and one oxygen atom (hydroxyls) attach themselves to carbon atoms (other compounds including phenols, acids, aldehydes, ketones, and esters, are also formed in this way). Ethyl alcohol, found in beers, wines, and liquors, is just one example. Alcohols generally tend to have good antiseptic and antiviral properties, as well as an uplifting quality. They are also usually non-toxic. They can be grouped into monoterpenols, sesquiterpenols, and diterpenols.

Monoterpenols

When a hydroxyl unit attaches itself to a terpene, the resulting alcohol is a monoterpenol. Those occurring in essential oils include menthol and linalool. These are strong bacteri-cides and combat infection. They are antiviral, stimulating, warming, and strengthening, and do not cause any skin irritation. Essential oils that are high in monoterpenols are some of the safest to use on children and the elderly.

Sesquiterpenols

A hydroxyl unit attaching to a sesquiterpene creates a sesquiter-penol. Oils high in sesquiterpenols can be good blood cleansers and tonics, and are nonirritant. Some have specific affinities to the heart or the liver.

Diterpenols

These are created when a hydroxyl unit is attached to a diterpene. These molecules are heavy and not very volatile, so only a few make it through the distillation process. Those that do have a structure resembling a human hormone and can have a balancing effect on the endocrine system.

PHENOLS

If a hydroxyl unit attaches itself to a ring of carbon atoms the resultant compound is called a phenol. In essential oils phenols are stronger than alcohols. They are powerful antiseptics and bactericides, and can often act as stimulants to the nervous and immune systems. Overuse may cause skin irritation.

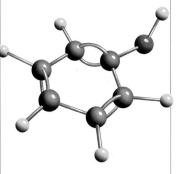

ABOVE *One phenol is also known as carbolic acid and was widely used as a disinfectant in World War I.*

ALDEHYDES

Aldehydes are formed by the oxida-tion of alcohols and often have a powerful aroma. In aromatherapy they tend to exhibit similar proper-ties to phenols or ketones, and can cause some skin irritation in sensi-tive people, though other compo-nents of the oil or another oil may prevent a reaction occurring. Citral, citronellal, and nerol are all impor-tant aldehydes, and are found in lemon-scented oils such as melissa, lemon balm, and lemongrass. Aldehydes can be anti-inflamma-tory, anti-infectious, tonic, hypoten-sive, and calming, and usually lower body temperature.

KETONES

In a ketone, a sole oxygen atom attaches itself to a carbon atom to form a unit that then joins with a hydrcarbon compound. A common ketone, though not a component in essential oils, is acetone (nail-varnish remover). Only a few ketones are present in any essential oil (none mentioned in this book contains a significant quantity) and many of them are neurotoxic. Used in moderation their effect is calming and sedative, and they can reduce fat, ease the flow of mucus, and encourage scar tissue formation. Ketones can also be digestive, anal-gesic, stimulant, or expectorant.

ACIDS AND ESTERS

Organic acids are very different from inorganic acids, and both acids and esters are complex combi-nations of carbon, hydrogen, and oxygen. Esters have a fruity aroma, can be anti-inflammatory and effec-tive for skin problems, and also have fungicidal properties. They have a balancing effect on the nervous system by being variously calming or uplifting as required. Acids in essential oils also have anti-inflammatory properties.

LACTONES

Lactone molecules tend to be too big to pass through the distillation process and so usually occur only in oils prepared by expression, or in concretes such as jasmine oil. Lactones tend to be useful in lower-ing temperature and alleviating catarrh, and seem to be the compo-nent of fruit oils that is responsible for skin photosensitivity.

Carrier Oils

A CARRIER OIL, *also called a base oil or plain oil, is a vegetable or nut oil that can be used to dilute essential oils for massage or in any other situation when the oil is to be applied directly to the skin. The essential oil disperses in the carrier, allowing a small quantity of the former to be spread over quite a large area of the body.*

ABOVE *Dilute essential oils in a carrier before use on the skin.*

Only good-quality vegetable oils should be used as carrier oils: cold-pressed oil is best, as it retains its vitamin and mineral content. A small quantity of a second, richer oil can also be added to the blend.

WHEATGERM OIL

• GENERAL DESCRIPTION: Rich in protein and in vitamins B and E.
• SPECIFIC USES: *In massage, wheatgerm oil is often used in a 10 percent dilution with another carrier oil to enrich, nourish, and preserve the skin. Its most common use is in pre-*serving aromatherapy formulae, when it is also used in a 10 percent dilution. The high vitamin E content of the oil acts as a preservative (antioxidant) and extends storage life from a few weeks to up to six months.

> ### CAUTION
> Do not use wheatgerm oil if you have a wheat allergy.

AVOCADO OIL

• GENERAL DESCRIPTION: Rich in vitamins A, B, and D all of which are good for skin problems. This is a viscous oil with a distinct odor and a green tint. For this reason avocado oil is best used in a 5 or 10 percent dilution with another carrier oil.

LEFT *Its higher vitamin content makes avocado oil ideal for problem skins.*

• SPECIFIC USES: *In dilution avocado oil is beneficial for skin problems. It is also suitable for people with wheat allergies who cannot use wheat based oils (see above).*

JOJOBA OIL

• GENERAL DESCRIPTION: This is not strictly an oil but a wax from the fruit of the desert plant *Simmondsia chinensis*. It is best used in 10 percent dilution with a carrier oil.
• SPECIFIC USES: *Useful for dry eczema and makes a good base for hair oil. It can be particularly beneficial for infantile eczema, cradle cap, and other dry skin complaints.*

WHEATGERM OIL

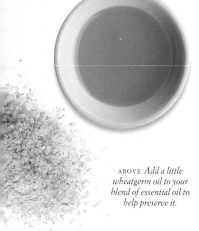

ABOVE *Add a little wheatgerm oil to your blend of essential oil to help preserve it.*

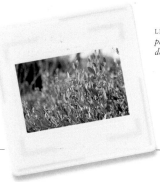

LEFT *The jojoba cactus plant grows wild in the deserts of North America.*

JOJOBA OIL

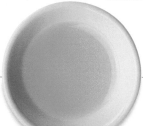

SOYA OIL
AND BEANS

SOYA OIL

- GENERAL DESCRIPTION:
A very nourishing and readily absorbed oil, soya oil is also ideal for people with wheat allergies (see wheatgerm oil).
- SPECIFIC USES: *This oil is valued (particularly in France) for its ability to lower cholesterol levels. High-quality soya oil can also be useful in massage for acne sufferers.*

Soya oil is an inexpensive, versatile oil, but be careful to choose only the purest oil of the finest quality, especially if you have sensitive skin.

APRICOT
KERNEL OIL

ABOVE *Peach and apricot oils are very versatile and may be used on all skin types.*

PEACH/APRICOT KERNEL OIL

- GENERAL DESCRIPTION: Very light, penetrating, and virtually odorless.
- SPECIFIC USES: *These oils can be used on all types of skin and are extremely nourishing.*

VITAMINS, MINERALS, AND FATTY ACIDS

Although beneficial to the skin itself, the minerals, vitamins, and essential fatty acids present in cold pressed carrier oils do not necessarily reach the body's internal systems. Vegetable oils frequently have larger molecules than essential oils and are often unable to pass through the skin.

Carrier oils vary greatly in quality. Unfortunately, organic carrier oils are quite rare. The use of pesticides and fertilizers in the normal production of oils severely reduces their mineral content. Cold pressing helps the oils to retain a significant quantity of the nutrient content of the original crops from which they are extracted. This process tends to involve temperatures of not more than 170° F (60° C). Oils that have not been cold pressed tend to have been subjected both to temperatures of over 392° F (200° C) and to solvent extraction.

Try to use the carrier oil that contains the properties best suited to your skin. Sweet almond oil contains vitamins A, B1, B2, and B6 and a small quantity of vitamin E. It also contains a high percentage of mono- and polyunsaturated fatty acids. Carrot oil is rich in beta-carotene, vitamins, B, C, D, and E and essential fatty acids. Used regularly, it is an effective skin rejuvenator so it is worth adding a small amount to skin creams that are used every day. Good quality sunflower oil contains vitamins A, B, D, and E and is high in unsaturated fatty acids. It can help bruises and skin diseases.

GRAPESEED OIL

- GENERAL DESCRIPTION: Grapeseed oil is very pure, high in polyunsaturates and extremely light. It is also very penetrating.
- SPECIFIC USES: *This oil has slightly astringent qualities and is therefore good for young skin. It is also beneficial for those who suffer from acne.*

CAUTION

Except in a first-aid situation, such as a wasp sting, a deep cut, a burst pimple, a domestic burn, or the prevention of a bruise, essential oils should never be used neat on the skin.

SWEET ALMOND OIL

- GENERAL DESCRIPTION: A good skin softener and lubricant.
- SPECIFIC USES: *This oil is usually tolerated well by sensitive skins and is also particularly good for dry or wrinkled skin. The essential oil of the bitter almond is not used in aromatherapy.*

SWEET
ALMOND OIL

ABOVE *Use sweet almond oil for sensitive, dry, or wrinkled skin.*

Blending

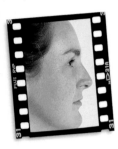

THERE IS MUCH *to be said for literally following your nose in creating a wide variety of blends with the oils. Remember that attractive-smelling oils can be used with more therapeutic oils to make a pleasing combination.*

LEFT *Follow your nose when selecting essential oils for home use and you won't go far wrong.*

Blending suggestions for each oil are included in the Materia Medica. You can experiment with these, but you can also simply follow your intuition.

Scientists have proved that when certain oils enter the bloodstream they head for, or have an affinity with, specific organs or systems of the body. Herbalists and healers knew this long before it was verified by successful scientific experimentation. Try it yourself: pick up a bottle of oil, inhale its aroma deeply, and ask yourself where in your body the oil wants to go or what it wants to do. When you then read about the oil, it is very likely you will discover that you have been scientifically accurate in your response. It is this intuition that you can use when creating your own blends.

It is important to use only a very small amount of essential oil in proportion to base oil, especially if you want to use the blend for a massage or skin preparation. If you add more essential oil than you

intended, or if either you or the person you are massaging doesn't like the smell you have created, rinse the blend away and start again. It may feel like a waste of oil, but this is where respecting the power of the oils and your instinctive reaction to them becomes very important. Saving a little bit of oil is not

worth the risk of skin irritation or other problems. Good proportions to use when blending the essential oils with each other or with carrier oils for use on the skin are given on the opposite page.

BELOW *Herbalists from the past knew which plants to pick to treat specific organs of the body.*

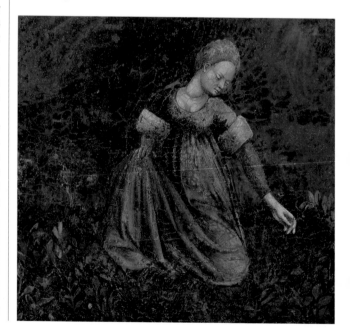

> **TIP**
> Always follow your instincts and throw away any blend that you or your partner finds offensive.

MASSAGE OIL

Allow six drops of essential oil to 3–4tsp. (15–20ml.) of carrier oil. A full-body massage on an adult requires approximately 4tsp. (20ml.) of oil. This will provide you with enough oil to allow your hands to slide smoothly over the skin without leaving your partner completely squelching in oil. If you start out in a massage with too little carrier oil but the right quantity of essential oil, add more carrier oil but no more essential oil.

Massage oils can be blended in the proportion 3–2–1 for a spread of high-, middle-, and base-note oils), or 2–2–2 for a mixture of middling oils. Only rarely do you need more than one drop of a base-note oil for a full-body massage – which is just as well as they are often the most expensive!

BELOW *Blend your essential oils with the carrier before beginning your massage.*

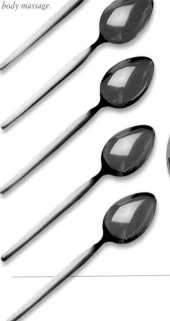

GENTLE HAND MASSAGE

TOWEL COVERING BODY

RELAXED PATIENT

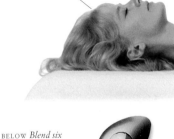

BELOW *Blend six drops of essential oil with 4tsp. of carrier oil to make a sufficient quantity for a full body massage.*

BATH OIL

The proportions for bath oil can be the same as for massage oil. It is fine to use only one or two oils, but in blending the sum can often be greater than the individual parts (this is called synergy). Three oils, therefore, often form the right balance for creating both a rich smell and a powerful blend.

CAUTION

Break up neat essential oils on the surface of your bathwater to prevent them burning your skin.

BELOW *Use up to three different oils to create an aromatic and powerful blend for the bath.*

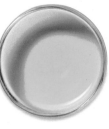

ATLAS CEDARWOOD OIL

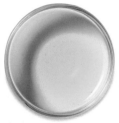

LEMONGRASS OIL

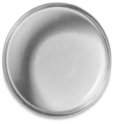

BERGAMOT OIL

Buying and keeping oils

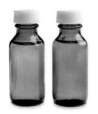

ABOVE *Keep your essential oils in air-tight containers that have a tight fitting screw-top lid.*

OILS CAN *vary a great deal in price and quality depending on both environmental and economic factors so it is worth while taking care over which oils you choose to purchase. Once bought, they should be stored carefully to ensure that they stay in good condition for as long as possible. Essential oils are the vital energies of naturally grown plants and should be treated with respect.*

WHERE TO BUY OILS

Essentials can be purchased from an oil shop, from a herbalist who stocks oils, from a mail-order distributor, or even from your local pharmacy or health-food store. Mail order is often a good bet and most firms seem to respond quickly. If you want a recommendation of a local supplier, ask an aromatherapist in your area or enquire at your local health center. You could also try telephoning an aromatherapy training school to find out which oils they recommend: they may even distribute their own.

BELOW *The plants used to make essential oils come from all over the world.*

KNOW YOUR LATIN

Knowledge of the Latin names is useful as it allows you to be certain exactly which oils you are buying. This is especially true if you are buying from a small company that sells relatively inexpensive oils and you are curious about the quality of their products.

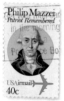

U.S.A.

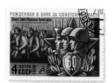

RUSSIA

PHILLIPINES

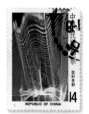

CHINA

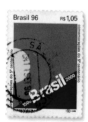

BRAZIL

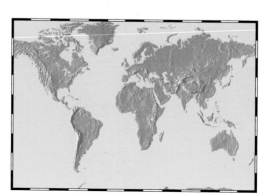

MALAYSIA

THE PRICE OF OILS

The price of individual oils varies quite a bit, but jasmine, rose, neroli, and melissa are usually the most expensive. Sometimes the price of oils can be affected by availability, dependent either on the politics of the country of origin or the success of the plant crop that year.

Variation in price can, of course, reflect the quality of the oil. For example, some very cheap jasmine oil is sold as essential oil, but it is likely to be either heavily adulterated or synthetic. The more expensive oils are also often blended with sweet almond oil, so despite appearances are not in fact pure.

Overall, the better the quality of the oil you buy, the greater will be its therapeutic powers. That said, a ⅛oz. (5ml.) bottle of many of the oils covered in this book need not be expensive, even if the oil is of good quality. And even if one or two are expensive, remember that you need so little, a bottle will probably last long enough to pay for itself.

> **CAUTION**
> Never leave a bottle of essential oil on a polished or painted surface as the chemicals in the oil could damage it.

KEEPING OILS

In ideal conditions essential oils may keep for six years or longer, although the average shelf life is probably about two years. Citrus oils do not have such a long life expectancy, and while they do last longer if kept in the refrigerator, they may become clouded.

Essential oils deteriorate in sunlight and, although blue bottles may look lovely, they let more sunlight through than bottles at the red end of the color spectrum. It is therefore best to keep your essential oils in a tightly sealed brown or amber bottle. If you do keep oils in blue bottles, you must place them in a cool, dark place.

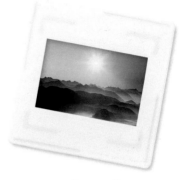

ABOVE *Keep your oils away from direct sunlight to preserve their shelf life.*

Remember also that essential oils are volatile by nature: not only will they vaporize, but the lighter molecules will disappear first, thereby changing the composition of the oil. To prevent this happening, ensure that your oil bottles have tight-fitting screwtop lids.

When essential oils are mixed into lotions, creams, or ready-made massage oils, the blend will last only as long as the carrier oil (probably around six months). Although the carrier will eventually go rancid, the effects of the essential oils will not be lost. Wheatgerm oil added to a homemade blend will help to preserve it (*see page 24*).

> **CAUTION**
> Absolutes and resinoids have a shorter life than distilled oils because over time they thicken and the smell of the solvent becomes more obvious.

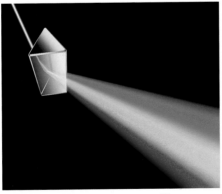

LEFT *This bottle may be pleasing to the eye but oils will keep better in brown bottles.*

ABOVE *Choose your bottles from the red end of the color spectrum to prevent fast deterioration.*

Homemade Preparations

EQUIPPED WITH *a stove and the simplest of kitchen utensils, it is possible to make an array of basic creams, lotions, room sprays, and aftershaves containing your favorite oils for yourself, your family, and friends. If you set aside an afternoon you can have a lot of fun and end up with something uniquely personal to show for it. Choose your oils well and you can create a homemade preparation that is both beautifying and therapeutic. Stir, blend, and enjoy!*

Any essential oils can be added to an unperfumed cream or lotion, selected according to skin type and usage. Only ten drops of essential oil are needed per 9fl. oz. (250ml.) bottle, and these drops can be taken from between one and three essential oils. Recipes for easy to make homemade toiletries are given below.

TONERS

Basic Recipe
*1tsp. (5ml.) vodka
5 drops in total of one or
two essential oils
4fl. oz. (100ml.) distilled
or filtered water*

Place the vodka and essential oils in a glass container with a lid and shake well. Top up the container with the water and shake again.

AFTERSHAVE

Increase the amount of vodka used in the basic recipe from 1tsp. to 2tsp. (10ml.). This will increase the astringency of the blend and make an effective or aftershave.

ROOM SPRAYS

For a refreshing room spray, double the quantity of the essential oils used in the basic toner recipe. Ensure that this spray is never used on your skin as it may cause irritation.

TALCUM POWDER

Any unscented talcum powder can be turned into an exotic, luxurious product with very little effort. Flower petals, such as roses or jasmine petals, can also be added as an attractive touch.

Place the unscented talc in a jar, add one or two drops from each of your chosen essential oil or oils (up to three), and shake well. Use from six to ten drops of oil for a small container of talc.

BATH SALTS

Use a good quantity of unscented bath salts and add two or three drops of each chosen oil (up to three oils). You can also add flower petals such as rose and chamomile to the blend. Relax and enjoy!

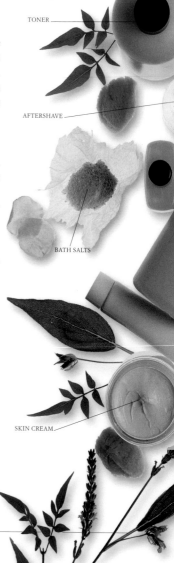

TALCUM POWDER

TONER

AFTERSHAVE

BATH SALTS

SKIN CREAM

RIGHT You can make a wide variety of homemade toiletries with very little effort or cost.

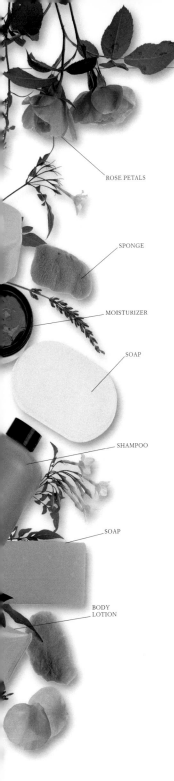

ROSE PETALS

SPONGE

MOISTURIZER

SOAP

SHAMPOO

SOAP

BODY
LOTION

SKIN CREAM

Ingredients
8fl. oz. (225ml.) carrier oil
8fl. oz. (225ml.) filtered water
1 stick of beeswax
¼ tsp. borax

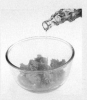

1 Put the beeswax in a heatproof bowl and pour in half the carrier oil. Place over a pan of boiling water to melt.

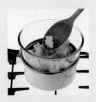

2 Dissolve the borax completely in 1tbsp. of boiling water and add to the hot oil and beeswax. Add the rest of the oil.

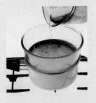

3 Add the filtered water to the mixture and beat until all the water has been incorporated. Allow the mixture to cool, then pot your cream.

AROMATIC SOAP

Ingredients
8fl. oz. (225ml.) carrier oil
8fl. oz. (225ml.) water
8–16fl. oz. (225–450ml.) pure, unscented vegetable soap flakes
3 essential oils

1 Place all the ingredients in a heatproof bowl over a saucepan of hot water and dissolve the soap flakes.

2 Remove the bowl from the heat and use a whisk to blend the ingredients.

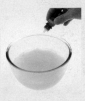

3 Allow to cool slightly, then add five drops each of three essential oils. Pot the soap and allow it to cool.

Aromatherapy for Modern Living

MANY PEOPLE turn to aromatherapy for no more specific reason than "stress relief." We put our bodies on "red alert" when there is no real danger present and then gradually drain away our bodies' resources to maintain ourselves in that condition. Aromatherapy is the perfect antidote to the stresses and strains of modern living.

Stress manifests itself physically in many ways, and many of the problems that people present to their physician or alternative therapist have their roots in stress. For example, chronic headaches or migraines, insomnia, backache, headaches, and stomach upsets are often the physical symptoms of stress. The use of aromatherapy oils in the home can be hugely beneficial in combating stress: relaxing in a warm aromatherapy bath or falling asleep while breathing a pleasant, relaxing aroma can bring nothing but beneficial results. If you know that your lifestyle is stressful, why not try to make time for yourself on a regular basis?

RIGHT *Essential oils may provide a useful and natural remedy for the tensions, disappointments, and pressures encountered in daily life.*

THE CAUSES OF STRESS

Aromatherapy oils can be a very powerful aid in coping with the physiological and emotional challenges of a stressful lifestyle. It is important to look at the causes of stress, which can lead to a wide range of problems, from insomnia to heart disease.

Physical Factors
• Lack of exercise results in stiffness, poor circulation, poor stamina, and low energy.
• Tension leads to insomnia, which in turn leaves you tired and preoccupied the next day and possibly having difficulty in sleeping the next night.
• Rushed meals and a bad diet can lead to both digestive problems and low vitality.

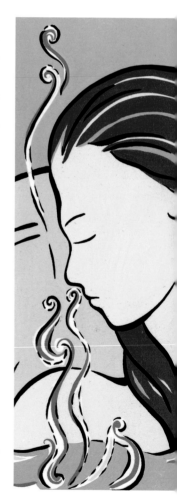

RIGHT *Surround yourself with calming aromas and discover a feeling of deep peace and relaxation.*

Environmental Factors

• Road rage in all its many manifestations and the stress that comes from public transport delays are traumatic. Remember that all the upsets you brush aside each day can come back to haunt you in the form of stress and its related illnesses.

• The quality of the air we breathe and the water we drink is crucial. Do you think about them, or are you unaware of their effects?

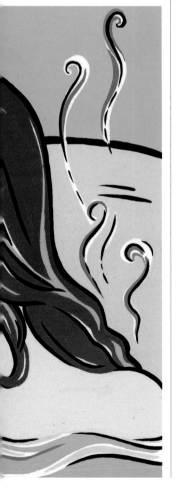

Emotional Factors

• Personal relationships can, sadly, be a great cause of stress, from the smallest domestic tiff to a divorce or children leaving home.

• Bereavement can cause a huge amount of grief and stress.

Mental Factors

• Money, or the lack of it, is the reason many people drive themselves too hard and spend too long at work. Like any other form of stress, this can deplete your body's resources and lead to illness.

• Job insecurity and dissatisfaction can be a major cause of stress, as can the struggle to get a job at all.

UNSATISFACTORY SOLUTIONS

In an effort to combat the problems of stress, many people turn to alcohol, drugs, cigarettes, or overeating.
But:

• Smoking can lead to chest, lung, and heart disease.

• Excessive alcohol can lead to high blood pressure, cirrhosis, hangovers, weight gain, as well as a whole host of emotional and relationship problems .

• Drug-taking can lead to serious addiction and a chemical imbalance in the body.

• Overeating can lead to weight gain, low self-esteem, apathy, and heart problems.

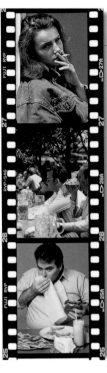

LEFT *Combat stress with essential oils – a safe and healthy alternative to smoking, drinking, or overeating.*

THE AROMATIC ALTERNATIVE

Aromatherapy can provide a healthy, successful alternative to all of the unsatisfactory solutions listed above. Essential oils can lift your mood and clear your head, as well as relieve pain and tension and ensure a good night's sleep. In the home environment, an aromatherapy bath can be very relaxing, while oils in a vaporizer can lift the mood and aid restful sleep. However, the soothing and nurturing touch of an aromatherapy massage, whether with a professional therapist or a partner at home, is probably the best way to beat stress. Refer to "The Art of Massage" *(see pp. 34–35).*

HOME USE

The use of aromatherapy oils at home is perfectly safe and very beneficial as long as you follow the guidelines set out in this book. Ensure that no oils are taken internally and do not apply any directly to the skin, except as outlined in the first-aid uses covered in "Aromatherapy in the Home" *(see pp. 128–129).* Experiment, blend, and enjoy!

The Art of Massage

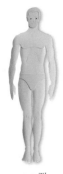

ABOVE *The benefits of massage can be felt on the whole body.*

THE COMBINATION *of aromatherapy and massage makes an ideal form of treatment as it works on both the body and the mind. An holistic massage takes into consideration the individual needs of the person receiving the massage, whether voiced on a verbal level or perceived on a spiritual level. With a little knowledge and experience, the essential oils can be blended with a carrier oil to provide a medium for massage that is both extremely beneficial for a person's health as well as a thoroughly relaxing and enjoyable event.*

Anyone can master the art of massage and everyone can benefit from it. It can improve circulation, aid good digestion, encourage respiration, and, by its effect on the lymphatic system, it can speed up the elimination of waste products from the body. This encourages the optimum functioning of the immune system. The combination of these physical benefits and the warm feeling of being cared for can encourage worries and stresses to fade away into the distance so that an aura of relaxation, peace, and well-being pervades the whole body. There are just a few basic massage strokes to learn. Everything else will only be variations of these.

BELOW *Any massage is more enjoyable if experienced in a comfortable room with a relaxing atmosphere.*

THE RIGHT ENVIRONMENT

If you are giving a massage at home it is important to create a comfortable environment, both for you and the person you are massaging.

First find a quiet, warm room: your partner will lose body heat quickly when he or she undresses, whereas you will probably get quite warm while you are doing the massage. Put some essential oil in a vaporizer to set the mood even if you will also be using essential oil on the skin during your massage.

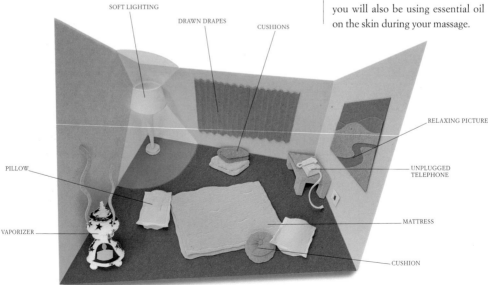

SOFT LIGHTING

DRAWN DRAPES

CUSHIONS

RELAXING PICTURE

PILLOW

UNPLUGGED TELEPHONE

MATTRESS

VAPORIZER

CUSHION

Turn the volume down on your answering machine and, if possible, turn off your telephone ringer. Let any other people in the house know what you are doing so that you won't be disturbed.

Some people enjoy massage to music while others prefer it without sound or an imposed rhythm. Try both and make your own decision. Subdued lighting can also aid the mood. Certainly bright lights shining in your partner's face, even if he or she has closed eyes, are not very relaxing.

Massaging on the floor should give both of you plenty of room. Pad the surface well with several blankets or a comforter for your partner, and make sure you have something soft to kneel on. Lots of pillows and towels are useful in allowing you to make your partner completely comfortable. Putting a pillow under your partner's knees when he or she is lying face up allows him or her to relax com-

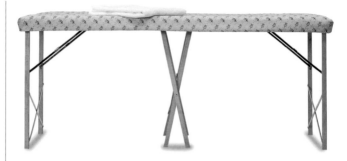

ABOVE *If you intend to massage your partner often, consider investing in a massage couch.*

pletely into the floor. If your partner is lying face down, experiment with pillows under the chest and ankles so the back can relax fully.

If you have a bad back or sore knees, you will probably find it easier to do the massage if your partner lies on a sturdy table. Some people have kitchen or dining tables that are both big enough and strong enough, and well-made pasting tables can also be good. Again, it is important to pad the surface of the table well. If you don't have an ideal table you might consider investing in a portable massage couch. Beds are too soft for massage: all the pressure you apply will be absorbed by the mattress, and the bed itself may well be at an awkward height.

It is important to keep your back straight and strong, and to use the weight of your body to give rhythm and support. If you are working at a table, keep your feet wide apart, bend your knees, and lean into your strokes. If you are on the floor, kneel with your knees apart or place one foot on the floor with the knee bent. Change position frequently.

THE RIGHT CLOTHES

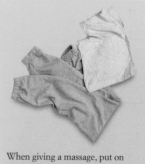

When giving a massage, put on loose-fitting, washable clothes (you may get oil on them) and either wear comfortable shoes or go barefoot. Remove all jewelry and watches as they may distract you and scratch your partner's skin. Also make sure that your nails are short and neat.

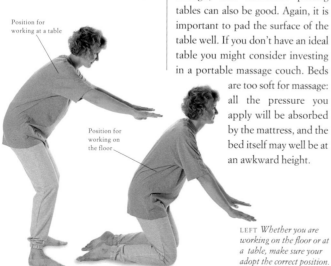

Position for working at a table

Position for working on the floor

LEFT *Whether you are working on the floor or at a table, make sure your adopt the correct position.*

Effleurage

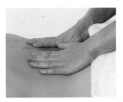

THIS IS THE *movement you will use most frequently as it is the basic stroking movement. This stroke encourages your partner to relax. You can do a few effleurage strokes on each part of the body before you put oil on your hands so that your partner becomes accustomed to the feel of your hands on his or her skin.*

TIP

It is best to apply firmer pressure as you slide up the body toward the heart, and to release the pressure as you come down the body away from the heart. Use enough oil for your hands to slide easily over the skin.

THE BACK

A good back massage is one of the pleasures of life. It is extremely relaxing and does much to alleviate stress and tense or painful muscles.

STEP 1
Start with your hands flat on the bottom of your partner's back.

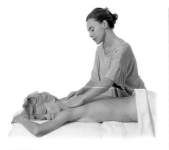

STEP 2
Gently slide your hands up the middle of the back, one on each side of the spine. Then fan your hand out over the shoulders, and round and down the sides of the body.

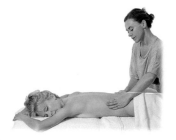

STEP 3
Take care not to drag the skin as you glide your hands lightly down the sides of the body back to the starting position. Repeat the stroke several more times.

STOMACH AND ABDOMEN

Effleurage is also very effective when performed in a clockwise direction on the stomach and abdomen: one hand describes a complete circle and stays in constant contact with the skin while the other describes a semicircle. Your hands cross as the full circle is completed.

THE LEG

Gentle stroking on the legs stimulates circulation, bringing blood and nutrients to the legs. It also stimulates the lymphatic system.

CAUTION
Do not apply pressure over the knee.

THE ARMS

Massaging the arms helps to reduce tension and promotes a feeling of deep relaxation.

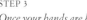

To perform effleurage on the arms, hold your partner's hand with one of yours and slide your other hand up and down their arm. You can concentrate on the tension in the upper or lower arm. Be careful to stroke gently over the inside elbow.

STEP 1

To perform effleurage on a leg, start with both hands at the foot, fingers pointing inward. Slowly glide them up the leg together, pressing on either side of the bone.

STEP 2

Glide your hands up together to the top of the thigh. Then fan your hands out and slowly bring them back down each side of the leg.

STEP 3

Once your hands are back in their original starting position, repeat the stroking movement again several more times.

Kneading

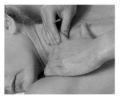

THIS MOVEMENT *is beneficial for the tops of the shoulders and the sides of the middle back, and for the fleshy areas of the thighs and the calves. This technique helps to relax the deeper muscles and improves the circulation, bringing in fresh blood and encouraging the elimination of waste products.*

STEP 1

Place your hands flat on the skin with your elbows pointing outward and your fingers pointing inward.

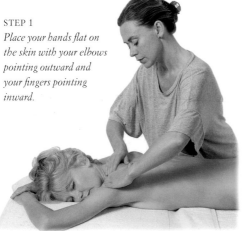

WRINGING

This technique adds a twist to the basic kneading movement to provide a deeper and more stimulating stroke. Place your hands side-by-side on the part of the body that you are massaging. Then grasp the flesh with both hands and start to work in opposite directions as if you are wringing out a cloth.

CAUTION

On less fleshy areas such as the upper arms, knead more lightly with the fingertips.

STEP 2

With one hand, gently but firmly take hold of a handful of flesh and push it toward the other hand.

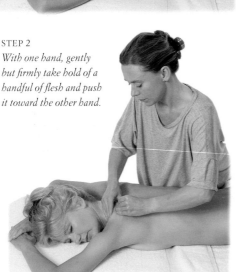

STEP 3

Then release the flesh and take it up in your other hand in the same way. Rhythmically grasp and release the flesh with alternate hands, one hand releasing the flesh as the other picks it up.

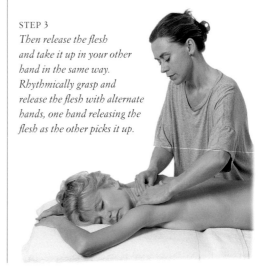

Thumb Pressures

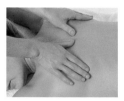

DEEP, DIRECT *thumb pressures or circles, called petrissage, are very beneficial if applied to the big muscles on either side of the spine, around the shoulders, and in a line up the middle of the back of the leg. They help to ease tension and are also very relaxing.*

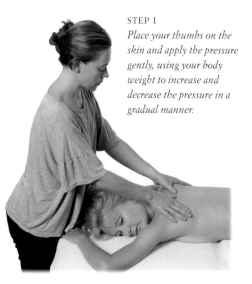

STEP 1

Place your thumbs on the skin and apply the pressure gently, using your body weight to increase and decrease the pressure in a gradual manner.

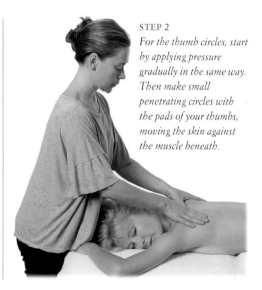

STEP 2

For the thumb circles, start by applying pressure gradually in the same way. Then make small penetrating circles with the pads of your thumbs, moving the skin against the muscle beneath.

PROBLEM AREAS

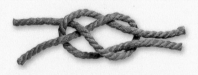

As you work you will probably discover tension somewhere in your partner's body that feels like stiffness, tautness, tenderness, or lumps under the skin. These "knots" are bunched-up muscles or toxins that can't yet escape the body. Apply pressure directly to the tense areas or work around the surrounding areas. Don't press too hard or too suddenly or you will hurt your partner and make him or her even more tense.

TICKLISH AREAS

Ticklishness is often caused by nervous tension. Try a little more pressure or alternatively work on the surrounding area and return to the ticklish area later, when it will probably have relaxed.

CAUTION

Avoid working directly on the spine or back of the knee.

Beginning the Massage

ONCE THE *essential oils have been chosen, the room has been prepared, and you feel ready to start, ask your partner to strip down to their underpants, or to remove all their clothes if you both feel happy about that. Blend the oils in a small bowl, rather than using them straight from a bottle. This way you can reach for more oil with one hand and maintain physical contact with your partner with the other.*

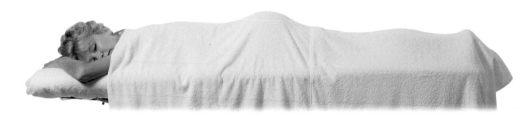

Before you begin, shake your hands, wring them out and rub them together to warm them if necessary. When your partner is in position, completely covered with towels, place your hands on his or her back or the soles of the feet, and breathe deeply. Take a moment to think how you would like your treatment to go, how you would like it to feel, and what you would like to be able to do for your partner. Then uncover the part of the body you want to work on first and oil your hands. You will soon learn how much oil to use, but always make sure you have enough to allow your hands to glide smoothly. Too much is better than too little, and you can always use a towel to dab off any excess – in any case, you should do this as you finish massaging each area of the body. Make the first contact with your partner's skin very gradually and gently. If you start the massage strongly and with no warning, your partner will get quite a shock. Use the effleurage stroke to oil your partner's body evenly, then use a combination of effleurage, kneading, and petrissage to massage each area of the body in turn. When you gain confidence you will find that the fun of massage lies in experimentation. A firm, strong massage will be invigorating and stimulating, while a slow, gentle massage will be completely relaxing. You should also make sure you get some massages yourself, as this will allow you to learn how certain strokes feel on the receiving end. If you do a lot of massage your hands will soon get strong, but if not, you can exercise them by squeezing a soft rubber ball or using Chinese exercise balls.

ABOVE *Make sure your partner is comfortable, warm, and completely covered in towels.*

BELOW *Each time you give a massage ask your partner what he or she would like.*

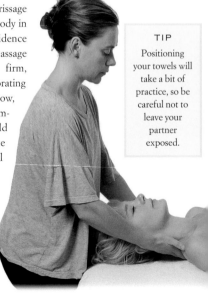

TIP

Positioning your towels will take a bit of practice, so be careful not to leave your partner exposed.

The Massage Sequence

THERE IS *no right or wrong order to carry out a massage, but many therapists choose to begin on the back when they are doing a full-body massage. The back is a good, large area to begin on and people very often hold tension either between their shoulders or at the base of their spine. Before beginning your massage check that your partner is warm and comfortable.*

THE SEQUENCE

An ideal massage sequence is as follows: back (1), back of legs (2), turn over, front of legs (3), arms (4), stomach (5) and chest, neck (6), scalp (7), and, lastly, the face (8).

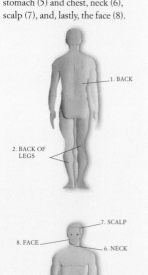

1. BACK

2. BACK OF LEGS

7. SCALP

8. FACE

6. NECK

4. ARMS

5. STOMACH

3. FRONT OF LEGS

STEP 1

Often the best way to begin a massage is with gentle relaxing effleurage to the whole of your partner's back. You will find that your partner will begin almost immediately to relax and enjoy the massage.

EFFLEURAGE THE WHOLE BACK

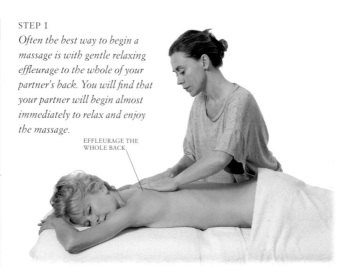

STEP 2

Either uncover legs one at a time or both together if you are confident that they will be warm enough.

KNEAD THE CALVES

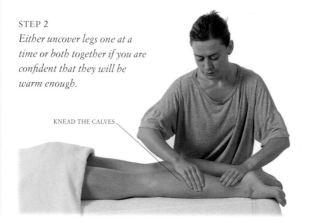

STEP 3

For the front of the legs focus your attention on kneading and effleuraging the fleshy thigh and work also on the feet. You can bend and circle the ankles, wiggle each toe, and stroke the sole and top of the foot with the length of your thumbs.

STROKE BOTH SIDES OF THE LEG

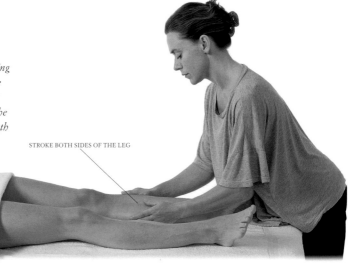

TIP
However inexperienced you are in massage, listen to your instincts and give the person you are massaging what you feel they need and you are likely to be right.

STEP 4

Massage each arm in turn. You can elevate the arm when you are holding your partner's hand to gain greater access to the upper arm. Work on the inside of the wrist with the length of your thumbs.

MASSAGE EACH ARM IN TURN

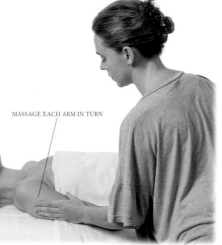

STEP 5

Remember to work exclusively clockwise on the stomach area as this is the direction of the digestive action. You can make gentle circles with your fingertips and circle your palms around your partner's belly button. Try to remember that this area is often quite sensitive.

WORK IN CIRCULAR MOVEMENTS

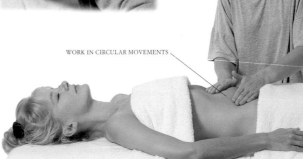

STEP 6

To massage the neck you can slide your hands under your partner's neck and work from there or you can gently lift and turn the head to one side, cradling the head in one hand while you use your other hand to massage the side of the neck that is exposed. You can also work on the back of the neck with your fingertips in that position.

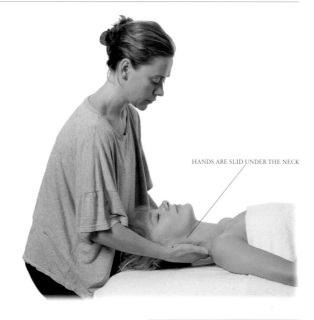

HANDS ARE SLID UNDER THE NECK

TIP

Be careful not to get oil (or your fingers) in your partner's eyes.

STEP 7

Massage the scalp above the forehead with your fingertips before moving on to do the face. Use effleurage strokes across and up the forehead and around the chin. You can use your third finger to make tiny petrissage circles around the cheekbones and out from the corners of your partner's mouth.

MASSAGE COURSES

Once you have mastered the basic strokes, it is well worth going on a short massage course run by a qualified teacher to improve your technique. You may find you want to train to be a professional therapist yourself and demonstrate to others the value of a caring, therapeutic touch.

USE YOUR FINGERTIPS
TO MASSAGE THE SCALP

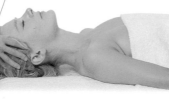

GENTLY STROKE THE FACE
TO FINISH THE MASSAGE

STEP 8

Finish the massage by gently resting your hands on your partner's head, cup them gently over their ears, or rest them on their shoulders.

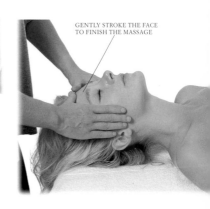

POINTS TO REMEMBER

• **Massage** should always be pleasurable, so encourage your partner to let you know what he or she particularly enjoyed or if anything was unpleasant or painful.

• **Rhythm** is the most important thing in a massage. If you vary the rhythms as you work, you will send waves of relaxation through your partner's body.

• **Once you get going**, try to keep one hand on the body throughout the massage. A good massage should feel like a single continuous stroke.

• **Vary your pressure.** It is best to start lightly, increasing the pressure when you feel that your partner has become accustomed to your touch on a particular area of his or her body, and then to finish lightly. Don't be afraid to work quite deeply over muscular areas such as the thighs and buttocks. Use your body weight to apply pressure.

• **Concentrate on the massage.** Don't let your mind wander and don't initiate conversation. If your partner wants to talk that's fine, but don't encourage it. You could suggest instead that you both concentrate on the physical sensations of the massage.

• **Don't forget to breathe** when you are giving a massage. When you are doing something new and concentrating hard, it is easy to hold your breath. Watch your partner's breathing, too. A good way to begin and end a massage is to ask your partner to take three deep breaths.

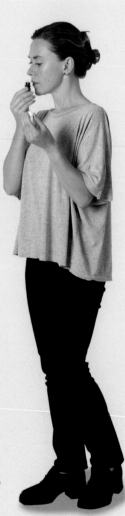

RIGHT *The person who gives the massage will usually enjoy the experience as much as the receiver.*

> ### TIP
> Remember to have a massage yourself sometimes – especially if you are working very hard.

If you want to know how deeply he or she is breathing, try matching your breathing rhythm to his or hers and see how it makes you feel. You can gently make your partner aware of his or her breathing at any time in the treatment, but be careful not to draw too much attention to it as your partner may become anxious. Ideally, your partner's breathing will relax and deepen naturally during the massage.

• **A full-body massage** usually takes up to 90 minutes. If you do not have this much time, concentrate on the areas that need massaging most; your partner can tell you which these are.

• **Don't take it too seriously** and don't worry. If you can't think what to do next just keep stroking the area you are working on with a full, relaxed hand, occasionally varying your rhythm. The ideas will come. You can give a pleasurable and therapeutic full-body massage just using effleurage.

A LOVING TOUCH

Remember that massage is a gift, not just for the receiver but for the giver as well. Touch is a two-way thing. The world would be a better place if we all gave and received a massage at least once a week.

HEALTH NOTES

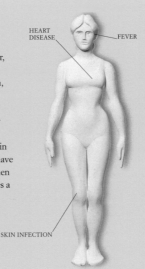

WHEN TO AVOID MASSAGE:

Do not massage anyone with the following conditions:

• High blood pressure or any heart problems, a contagious disease, a fever, or a high temperature.

• A skin infection, acute inflammation, or serious bruising.

• An inflammatory condition of the circulatory system such as phlebitis or thrombosis.

• Acute back pain, especially if the pain shoots down the arms or legs. If you have started massaging and this happens then stop and suggest that your partner sees a physician.

HEART DISEASE

FEVER

SKIN INFECTION

RIGHT *Certain medical conditions mean that massage is not advisable.*

IN ADDITION:

• Do not massage over varicose veins.

• Do not massage anyone who is diabetic or who has particularly high or low blood pressure without permission from his or her physician.

• Massage a person who is epileptic only if you are both extremely confident that you know how to cope with a fit if he or she should have one during the massage.

• (*see below* for massage during pregnancy).

CAUTION

Do not massage if you are unwell, lacking in energy, or if either of you have just eaten a big meal.

MASSAGE DURING PREGNANCY

Beyond the four-month stage massage can be wonderfully beneficial for pregnant women though it is not recommended before this time. A pregnant partner probably won't be comfortable lying on her front, so make her comfortable lying on one side or on her back and improvise. You can offer her extra pillows to put between her legs or to rest her bump on while she lies on her side, and then you can massage whatever bits you can get to. You can also give a wonderful back massage if you ask your partner to sit back to front on an upright chair leaning on the backrest.

CAUTION

Do not massage your partner if she is less than four months pregnant.

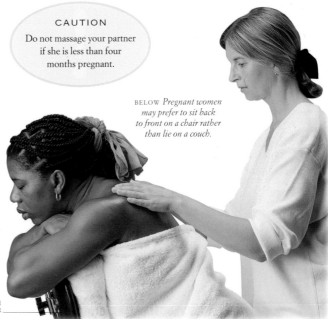

BELOW *Pregnant women may prefer to sit back to front on a chair rather than lie on a couch.*

LEAN AGAINST AN UPRIGHT CHAIR

Materia Medica

THIS SECTION *of the book contains profiles of 36 of the oils most commonly and safely used in aromatherapy. In each case, the plant from which the particular essential oil is derived is illustrated in color and fully described, together with a map that shows the principal areas in which it grows. A*

ANGELICA

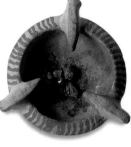

FRANKINCENSE

Properties box details the properties and aroma of each oil, as well as the way in which it is prepared or extracted from the source plant, its chemical constituents, fragrance note, and the other essential oils with which it can be blended to make a suitable and pleasing combination.

Many aromatherapy oils, and the plants from which they are derived, have been in use for literally thousands of years, and for each oil the variety of uses to which it has been put, and the beliefs and practices that have grown up around it, are fully described in a list of Uses Through the Ages. In a Health Notes box, the positive effects that each oil has upon the skin are given, along with the beneficial influences that each can have on our psychological well-being and emotional balance.

SWEET MARJORAM

GERANIUM

Essential oils can be used in a variety of ways, and in the Home Use panel a system of symbols (see opposite) highlights the best and most effective way to use each oil.

The oils are very therapeutic in respectful hands but can have powerful negative forces in ignorant or disrespectful hands. Warnings accompany any oil that should be used with caution, and these warnings should be taken to heart.

LEFT *The 36 plants described in this section are fully illustrated in color throughout to make identification easy.*

How to Use this Section

All aromatherapy oils are derived from plants. Materia Medica catalogues the plants that are the sources of the principal oils, and these plants are presented by their botanical names in alphabetical order. If you do not know the genus name of the source plant, the index at the back of the book will guide you to the particular plant or oil by its common name. Each entry is organized in the same way, as shown below, so that you can quickly find the information that you are looking for.

KEY TO DIFFERENT TECHNIQUES

Each oil is best used in particular ways; this system of symbols is used in each Home Use panel to provide a quick guide.

MASSAGE BATHS COMPRESS

INHALATION VAPORIZER FIRST AID

Each plant entry is organized in the same way for ease of reference. The left-hand page provides a general introduction to the plant, what it looks like and where it grows, and describes the properties of the oil, and the way in which it is extracted. The right-hand page gives details about the uses of the oil, and its historical importance, together with specific health notes.

Principal use for home aromatherapy. Symbols indicate the effective techniques.

Health Notes panel details the effects on the skin, and the psychological and emotional uses.

Full-color photograph of the plant growing in its natural situation.

Historical beliefs, myths, and practices concerning the particular plant.

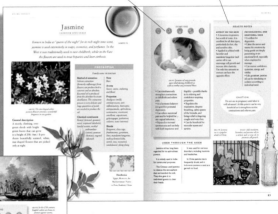

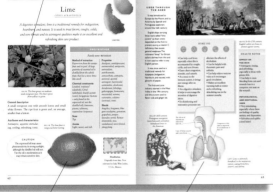

Close-up photograph of the plant matter from which the oil is derived.

Illustration of the physical effects and benefits of the aromatherapy oil.

PROPERTIES OF THE OILS

It has been observed that certain chemical constituents occur in a number of oils that display the same properties, and also that oils of the same botanical family have similar attributes and characteristics. A total of 21 botanical families provide the oils used in aromatherapy, and of these 16 yield the most well-known oils. The terms that describe the properties of the oils are fully explained in "Properties of Essential Oils" (*see p. 138*).

Yarrow

ACHILLEA MILLEFOLIUM

This healing plant has long been considered sacred by peoples all over the world. The Druids used it to foretell the weather, while in China the straight dried stalks are still used in I Ching divination. It has beneficial effects on the circulatory and digestive systems, as well as helping digestion and disorders of the intestine.

YARROW
LEAF

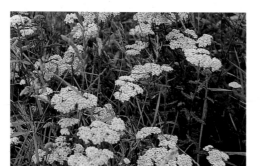

ABOVE *The powerful healing yarrow plant grows best in a sunny site.*

PROPERTIES

Family name **COMPOSITAE.**

Method of extraction
Steam distillation from dried flower heads.

Chemical constituents
Borneol (alcohol); cineole (ketone); azuline (sesquiterpene); limonene, pinene (terpenes).

Note
Top.

Aroma
Sweet and spicy.

Properties
Anti-inflammatory, antiphylogistic, antipyretic, antirheumatic, antiseptic, antispasmodic, astringent, carminative, cholagogue, cicatrisant, digestive, diuretic, expectorant, febrifuge, hemostatic, hypotensive, stimulant, stomachic, tonic.

Blends
Angelica, Atlas cedarwood, clary sage, juniper, lemon, melissa/lemon balm, Roman chamomile, rosemary, Scotch pine, vetiver.

General description

Balancing, grounding, hormone balancing, revitalizing, tonic for the nervous system. It can normalize mildly high blood pressure.

Attributes and characteristics

A smallish common herb with feathery leaves and pink and white flowers.

CAUTION

Excessive use may cause headaches and irritate sensitive skin in some individuals. As it is a very potent oil, use with care during pregnancy.

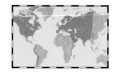

Distribution
Europe, west Asia,
North America.

LEFT *The yarrow plant can grow up to 3ft. (1m.) high. Small clusters of pinkish-white flowers appear from summer to autumn.*

USES THROUGH THE AGES

The name yarrow is a corruption of its old Anglo-Saxon name of gearwe, while the species name millefolium means "thousand leaves."

Legend has it that Achilles, warrior of the Iliad, used the plant to cure fellow soldier Telephos during the wars with Troy – hence the genus name.

The plant was once used as a charm in Scotland because it was thought to ward off evil spirits.

It was considered a sacred plant in ancient China and is used to read the I Ching, the ancient Chinese tool of divination.

In Chinese medicine it is thought to represent the perfect balance between natural opposites of yin and yang that manifest themselves as the polarities of hard and soft, hot and cold, wet and dry, and so on.

One of many folknames is "devil's plaything."

Young girls in Europe used to place it under their pillows in the hope that they would dream of their husband-to-be.

It was used both by Anglo-Saxons and crusaders to heal battle wounds delivered by iron weapons.

Yarrow is reputed to have a wide range of healing properties, and is traditionally used variously to treat lung cancer, epilepsy, hysteria, and diabetes.

In Norway it is used for rheumatism.

In Sweden it is added to beer.

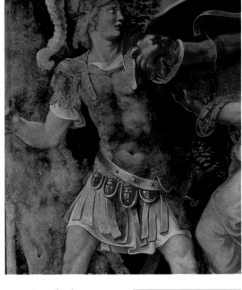

ABOVE *Legendary hero Achilles used the yarrow plant to heal a soldier after battle.*

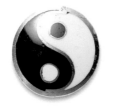

LEFT *The Chinese believe that the yarrow plant represents perfect balance, as in the yin/yang symbol.*

HOME USE

• As a general fortifier it acts on the bone marrow and stimulates corpuscle replacement.
• Can normalize mildly high blood pressure.
• Can help with varicose veins, chilblains, and other circulatory disorders, but you must not massage directly over the affected area.

• Balances irregular or heavy periods, and can help with inflamed ovaries, a prolapsed uterus, and fibroid discomfort.
• As an aid to good digestion, it can help to settle a nervous stomach, encourage the secretion of digestive juices, and improve nutrient absorption.
• Can also help with

diarrhea, flatulence, cramp, and colic.
• Encourages healthy perspiration by opening the sweat glands, and can help to cool a fever and clear a stuffy head.
• Has a balancing effect on urine flow, and helps to cure bedwetting.
• Alleviates muscle pain and headaches.

Angelica

ANGELICA ARCHANGELICA

Linked by name and legend to the Archangel Raphael, angelica has strong connections with the Christian Church and has long been used as a protective power against evil. Many parts of this large plant are utilized to provide pain relief and to stimulate the immune system.

ANGELICA
OIL

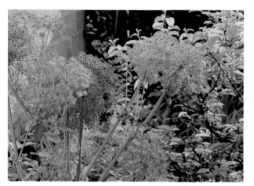

ABOVE *With its large, glossy, bright green leaves, the angelica plant can give any garden a lush tropical feel.*

PROPERTIES

Family name APIACEAE (UMBELLIFERAE).

Method of extraction
Steam distilled from the roots, rhizomes, fruit, and seeds of the plant.

Chemical constituents
Borneol, linalool (alcohols); bergaptene (lactone); limonene, phellandrene, pinene (terpenes).

Note
Base.

Aroma
Earthy, sweet, and penetrating.

Properties
Antispasmodic, aphrodisiac, carminative, depurative, diuretic, emmenagogue, expectorant, febrifuge, hepatic, nervine, stimulant, stomachic, sudorific, tonic.

Blends
Clary sage, geranium, grapefruit, lavender, lemon, mandarin/ tangerine, patchouli, Roman chamomile, sweet basil, vetiver.

General description

A large, hairy plant with fern-like leaves and greenish-white aromatic flowers.

Attributes and characteristics

Angelic, cleansing, comforting, elevating, revitalizing, stimulant, supportive.

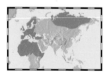

Distribution
Cultivated in Belgium, Hungary, Germany. Native to North Africa, Europe, Siberia. First found in Europe in the 16th century.

RIGHT *Growing up to 8ft. (2.4m.) high, angelica is an impressive plant.*

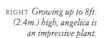

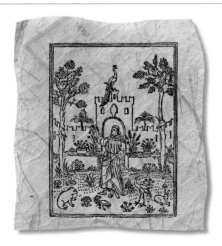

USES THROUGH THE AGES

🜚 It has been used in mystic rituals. The yellow juice from the roots was used in remedies to protect against the evil powers of witches.

🜚 It was grown in monasteries under the name of angel grass and has also been known as "herb of the Holy Spirit" or "herb of the Holy Ghost."

🜚 Legend has it that the virtues of angelica were revealed to a 10th-century monk by the Archangel Raphael in a dream so that it could be used as an antidote to the terrible effects of the plague. "Angelica water" is mentioned in a pamphlet published by the Royal College of Physicians in 1665, the year of the Great Plague.

🜚 It is often used to flavor the liqueurs Chartreuse and Benedictine, and is also an ingredient of gin and perfume.

🜚 Candied angelica is used as a cake decoration.

HOME USE

• Inhale it to counteract dizziness, nausea, and anxiety, and to clear congestion of the nose and help with chesty coughs, feverish colds, chronic bronchitis, and pleurisy.
• Can relieve indigestion, flatulence, nausea, and colic.
• Stimulates the lymphatic system, speeding up the healing of cuts and bruises and soothing sore and aching joints and muscles.
• Relieves cystitis through its antiseptic properties and its affinity with the urinary system. It can be used for rheumatic inflammation.
• Limits uric acid and so can benefit arthritis, gout, and sciatica.
• Is a rapid pain reliever and can help to relieve headaches, migraines, and toothache.

ABOVE LEFT *Known as the herb of the Holy Spirit, angelica was commonly grown in monasteries.*

RIGHT *Use of angelica helps boost the immune system and speeds up the healing of cuts and bruises.*

CAUTION

Angelica root oil may be phototoxic: avoid sunbathing and sunbeds after use or it may irritate the skin. It is also best to avoid it in pregnancy or if you are diabetic. Excessive use of angelica oil may act as a narcotic and slow down circulation.

HEALTH NOTES

EFFECT ON THE SKIN
• A good skin tonic. It can be helpful for dull and congested skin, as well as any skin eruption or irritant, including psoriasis.

PSYCHOLOGICAL AND EMOTIONAL USES
• Stimulates the nervous system and can help with exhaustion and stress.
• Promotes a feeling of balance and can give support to those facing difficult problems and decisions.
• Can aid meditation by making the user more open to angelic energies.

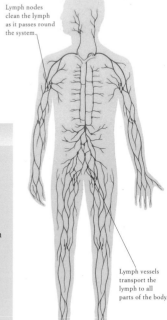

Lymph nodes clean the lymph as it passes round the system.

Lymph vessels transport the lymph to all parts of the body.

ROSEWOOD OIL

Rosewood

ANIBA ROSAEODORA

Best known for its use in the perfume industry and as a fine wood in furniture making, rosewood is also very beneficial as a skin care product. Use it sparingly, however, as its cultivation contributes to the deforestation of the Amazon rainforest.

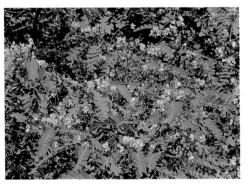

ABOVE *The rosewood is a medium-sized evergreen tree that grows in the Amazonian rainforest.*

PROPERTIES

Family name **LAURACEAE.**

Method of extraction
Steam distilled from heartwood chippings.

Chemical constituents
Geraniol, linalool, nerol, terpineol (alcohols); cineole (ketone); dipentene (terpene).

Note
Base.

Aroma
Warm, spicy, sweet, floral, and woody.

Properties
Analgesic, anticonvulsive, antidepressant, antimicrobial, antiseptic, aphrodisiac, bactericidal, cephalic, deodorant, insecticidal, stimulant (immune system), tonic. Also a cellular stimulant and tissue regenerator.

Blends
Atlas cedarwood, frankincense, geranium, patchouli, neroli, rose, rosemary, sandalwood.

General description

A tropical, evergreen tree with a reddish bark and heartwood, and yellow flowers.

Attributes and characteristics

It is deeply relaxing without being a sedative, and is a stimulant to the immune system. It is an aphrodisiac and is excellent for skin care.

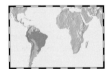

Distribution
Brazil (where it is known as jacaranda), Peru.

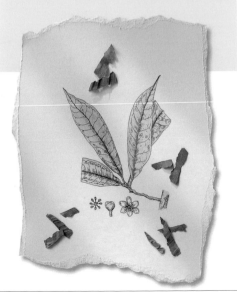

RIGHT *Rosewood essential oil is distilled from the heartwood chippings.*

HOME USE

• Boosts the immune system and helps the body to deal with viruses, infections, and chronic complaints.
• Is helpful against colds and fevers, and is good for ticklish coughs.
• Relieves headaches, especially if they are accompanied by nausea.

• Good for jetlag.
• A good deodorant as it balances excess moisture in the body.
• An insect repellent.
• A good tonic without having a particularly stimulant or sedative effect.

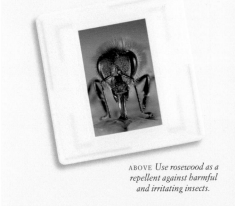

ABOVE *Use rosewood as a repellent against harmful and irritating insects.*

USES THROUGH THE AGES

꿎 Long established in perfumery, rosewood has only very recently been introduced into aromatherapy.

꿎 The Amazon Indians use it in the healing of wounds and for skin complaints.

꿎 The wood has been used in French cabinet-making and other building and carving, as well as in handles for domestic utensils such as brushes and knives.

꿎 Much rosewood now goes to Japan to make chopsticks and to the U.S.A. for furniture.

꿎 As the trees grow wild in the rainforest of Brazil there has been some concern about the excessive demand for the wood and oil causing damage to the environment. As a result, the Brazilian government now requires a new tree to be planted for every one cut down. This reafforestation is not proving successful, however, as the condition of the soil deteriorates once the primary forest is cut.

CHOPSTICKS

ABOVE *The Japanese use rosewood for making chopsticks.*

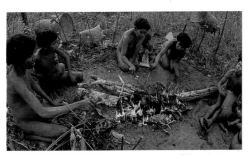

ABOVE *The Native peoples of the Amazonian rainforest use rosewood to treat skin complaints and heal wounds.*

HEALTH NOTES

EFFECT ON THE SKIN
• A cell stimulant and tissue regenerator, so is beneficial for acne and scars, aging skin, and wrinkles.
• Useful for cuts and wounds.
• Good for dry, dull, sensitive, combination, or inflamed skin.

PSYCHOLOGICAL AND EMOTIONAL USES
• Balances and calms the mind through its stabilizing effect on the central nervous system.
• Uplifting and reviving.
• Beneficial if you are feeling low, weary, or overburdened with problems, and is helpful with nervous tension and all stress-related conditions.

• Clears the head and steadies the nerves.
• An aphrodisiac and restores libido. It can help with impotence and frigidity, especially if the causes are emotional.
• A valuable oil to burn during meditation as it is very calming yet does not encourage drowsiness.
• An intimate, deeply relaxing oil.

CAUTION

Treat rosewood with respect – its use continues to contribute to the demise of the Amazon rainforest unless a solution can be found to aid reafforestation.

Frankincense

BOSWELLIA CARTERI

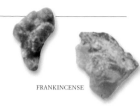

FRANKINCENSE

At one time valued as highly as gold, frankincense has been held in high regard for thousands of years. It is burned as an offering incense during the Catholic mass, and is also used to treat a wide range of conditions including nervous complaints and urinary tract infections.

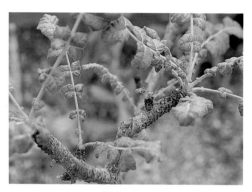

ABOVE *The frankincense tree yields a natural oleo-gum resin from its trunk.*

RIGHT *Frankincense oil is extracted by steam distillation from the oleo-gum resin.*

General description

Small tree or shrub with abundant pinnate leaves and white or pink flowers.

Attributes and characteristics

Cephalic, preservative, spiritual, uplifting, warming. It is also an aid to meditation.

PROPERTIES

Family name BURSERACEAE.

Method of extraction
Steam distillation from gum resin gathered from an incision in the bark.

Chemical constituents
Olibanol (alcohol); cadinene (sesquiterpene); camphene, dipentene, pinene, phellandrene (terpenes).

FRANKINCENSE OIL

Note
Base.

Aroma
Warm, rich, and slightly lemony. Long lasting and penetrating.

Properties
Anti-inflammatory, antiseptic, astringent, carminative, cicatrisant, cytophylactic, digestive, diuretic, emmenagogue, expectorant, sedative, tonic, uterine, vulnerary.

Blends
Bergamot, geranium, grapefruit, lavender, mandarin/tangerine, melissa/lemon balm, lime, neroli, patchouli, sandalwood, Scotch pine, sweet basil, vetiver.

CAUTION

Nontoxic, nonirritant, and non-sensitizing. However, use only in moderation, as you would any essential oil.

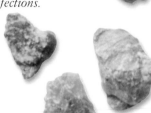

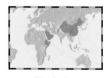

Distribution
Somalia, Ethiopia, China, Arabia.

USES THROUGH THE AGES

Frankincense has been revered for at least the last 3,000 years.

It has been burned in many cultures to appease the gods, and was one of the gifts from the three Magi to the infant Jesus.

At one time its commercial value was almost as great as gold.

It is still used as an offering incense during the Catholic mass.

It has been used by many cultures to treat almost every ailment, and has been burned to free the sick of evil spirits and to purify both the body and the soul.

The ancient Egyptians used it in cosmetics for face masks and in the embalming process. The Chinese used it to treat tuberculosis of the lymph glands and leprosy.

Frankincense means "real incense" in French.

The oil has another ancient name, olibanum, which means "oil from the Lebanon."

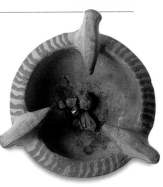

RIGHT *Frankincense has been used since ancient times as an incense.*

BELOW LEFT *The Three Kings offer frankincense to the newly born baby Jesus as a gift.*

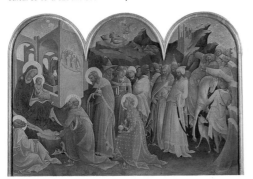

HOME USE

• Has a powerful effect on the mucus membranes, and is particularly effective in clearing the lungs and nasal passages.
• Can ease shortness of breath and promote good respiration.
• Its calming effect means that it is useful to inhale, particularly in stressful situations such as an asthma attack.
• Can help relieve indigestion.

• Has an affinity with the genito-urinary tract and can ease the discomfort of cystitis.
• A tonic to the uterus and can help regulate heavy periods.
• Very beneficial if used in the bathwater during menstruation or during pregnancy.
• Valuable in labor for its calming and focusing effects.

HEALTH NOTES

EFFECT ON THE SKIN
• Very valuable for use on aging skin as it has a tonic and regenerative effect.
• Its astringent qualities may help oily skins.
• Can assist in the healing of wounds and sores.

PSYCHOLOGICAL AND EMOTIONAL USES
• Beneficial in lifting the mood.
• Has a tonic effect on the nervous system yet also slows the breathing, and it has a calming, soothing, and elevating effect on the mind.
• Brings reassurance when you are lacking confidence or suffering emotional turmoil.

• Its use helps to break emotional commitments to the past and encourages personal and spiritual growth.
• Aids all kinds of meditation as it creates an elevated atmosphere.
• When it is burned it gives off trahydro-cannabinole, a consciousness-expanding chemical.

BELOW *Inhale frankincense oil from a handkerchief to bring relief to blocked nasal passages.*

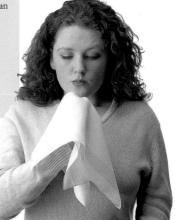

Ylang-Ylang

CANANGA ODORATA

A beautifully scented tree, the ylang-ylang is also known as the "perfume tree." During the Victorian era, it was used to make the hair oil known as macassar. It is calming and soothing and can be regarded as the "smelling salts" of aromatherapy.

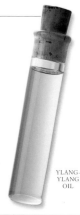

YLANG-
YLANG
OIL

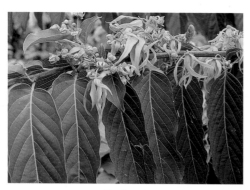

ABOVE *The ylang-ylang tree grows in tropical Asia, particularly Indonesia and the Philippines.*

PROPERTIES

Family name **ANNONACEAE**

Method of extraction
Steam distillation from fresh flowers. There are several grades of oil, extra superior being the best and most costly. The oil produced the first time the plant matter passes through the distillation process is the finest quality. Manufacturers then redistill to glean every possible drop of oil.

Chemical constituents
Benzoic (acid); farnesol, geraniol, linalool (alcohols); benzyl acetate (ester); eugenol, safrole (phenols); cadinene (sesquiterpene); pinene (terpene).

Note
Base.

Aroma
Floral and exotic.

Properties
Antidepressant, anti-infectious, antiseborrheic, antiseptic, aphrodisiac, euphoric, hypotensive, nervine, regulator, sedative (nervous), stimulant (circulatory), tonic.

Blends
Bergamot, grapefruit, jasmine, lavender, lemon, melissa/lemon balm, neroli, patchouli, rose, rosewood, sandalwood. The oil becomes more powerful when used in combination with others.

General description

A small, semiwild, tropical evergreen tree with brittle wood, shiny leaves, and pink, mauve, and yellow flowers. The yellow flowers produce the best oil.

Attributes and characteristics

Aphrodisiac, calming, euphoric, narcotic, soothing. Can lower high blood pressure when this is caused by stress or shock.

RIGHT *The ylang-ylang tree grows up to 68ft. (20m.) high and has fragrant pink, mauve, or yellow flowers.*

Distribution
Philippines, Java, Sumatra, Madagascar, Réunion.

HOME USE

- Lowers blood pressure and relaxes the central nervous system.
- Can help those suffering from palpitations.
- Balances the hormones and has an affinity with the reproductive system.
- As a uterine tonic it may be supportive on many physical, psychological, and emotional levels after a cesarian delivery.

- Helps with postnatal depression.
- As an intestinal antiseptic it can help with stomach upsets and mild or suspected food poisoning (put it in a burner or apply via gentle stomach massage).

CAUTION

It is best not to use it on inflamed skin or skin affected by dermatitis. Over-indulgence may bring on headaches and nausea.

USES THROUGH THE AGES

The name means "flower of flowers" and comes from the Malay alang ilang which refers to flowers that flutter in the breeze.

The tree is also called the "perfume tree."

In the Pacific women use oil of ylang-ylang on their hair in a blend with coconut oil, as a body moisturizer, and to avoid fever and infection.

It was an ingredient of macassar, a hair oil popular in 19th-century Europe

(antimacassars were subsequently invented to prevent the oil from staining chairbacks).

In Indonesia it is customary to spread a newly married couple's bed with ylang-ylang petals.

In the early 20th century researchers discovered that the oil could be effective against malaria, typhus, and intestinal infections. They also recognized the calming effect it has on the heart.

HEALTH NOTES

EFFECT ON THE SKIN
- Regulates sebum production and is good for both oily and dry skin conditions.
- A tonic for the scalp, it can encourage hair growth.

PSYCHOLOGICAL AND EMOTIONAL USES
- Very beneficial for emotional or physical difficulties that are connected to a lack of confidence.
- Calms excitement and hysteria, and it regulates adrenaline.

- Good for panic, anxiety, fear, and irritation and encourages a relaxed approach to problems and situations.
- Calms anger and frustration.
- Is an aphrodisiac and allays anxiety.
- In its first-aid application it is sniffed from the bottle like smelling salts, but if the symptoms persist you should consult your physician.

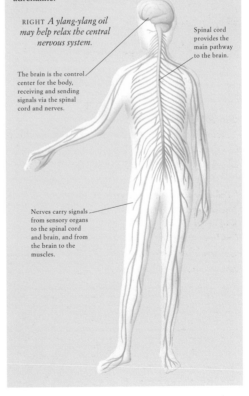

RIGHT *A ylang-ylang oil may help relax the central nervous system.*

Spinal cord provides the main pathway to the brain.

The brain is the control center for the body, receiving and sending signals via the spinal cord and nerves.

Nerves carry signals from sensory organs to the spinal cord and brain, and from the brain to the muscles.

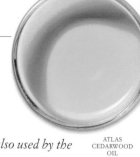

Atlas cedarwood

CEDRUS ATLANTICA

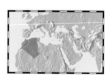

ATLAS
CEDARWOOD
OIL

Highly valued as a building wood, the Atlas cedarwood was also used by the Ancient Egyptians in cosmetics and perfumery as well as for embalming purposes. It has long been associated with spiritual occasions and is still used as an incense in present-day Tibetan temples.

CEDARWOOD CONE

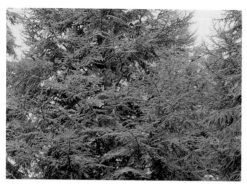

ABOVE *This large evergreen tree is native to the Atlas mountains of Algeria, but the essential oil comes mainly from Morocco.*

PROPERTIES

Family name **PINACEAE**

Method of extraction
Steam distillation from the wood. A resinoid and absolute can also be produced in small quantities.

Chemical constituents
Cedrol (alcohol); cadinene, cedrene, cedrenol (sesquiterpenes).

Note
Base.

Aroma
Like a dry sandalwood mixed with turpentine, and reminiscent of a freshly sharpened pencil.

Properties
Antiputrefactive, antiseborrheic, antiseptic, aphrodisiac, astringent, diuretic, emollient, expectorant, fungicidal, insecticidal, mucolytic, sedative (nervous), stimulant (circulatory), tonic.

Blends
Bergamot, clary sage, cypress, frankincense, jasmine, juniper, lavender, lemon, neroli, Roman chamomile, rose, rosemary, rosewood, vetiver, ylang-ylang.

General description

Pyramid-shaped evergreen tree with majestic stature. It can grow to a height of 120ft. (35m.). The wood is strongly scented because of the quantity of essential oil that it contains.

Attributes and characteristics

Antidepressant, aphrodisiac, elevating, grounding, protective, strengthening. Helps with hair loss and cystitis. Good for meditation.

RIGHT *Growing to a height of 120ft. (35m.), the Atlas cedarwood is an evergreen tree.*

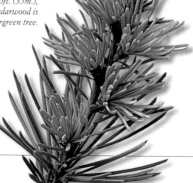

CAUTION
The oil is nontoxic, nonirritant and nonsensitizing. However, it is best avoided during pregnancy.

Distribution
Originally thought to come from the Lebanon and Cyprus, but named for the Atlas Mountains of Algeria. Today the finest oils come from Morocco.

HOME USE

• Can act as an expectorant and decongestant.
• Helps to alleviate the symptoms of bronchitis and catarrh.
• Has an affinity with the genito-urinary system and so can be beneficial for cystitis and similar conditions.
• Encourages the drainage of lymph and stimulates the breakdown of accumulated fats.
• Has a diuretic action and can help with cellulite, edema, and excess fat. Do not use it internally.

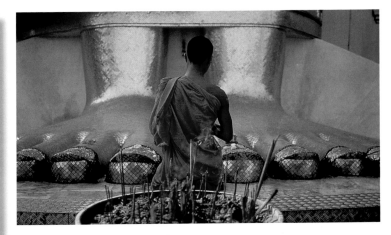

USES THROUGH THE AGES

❧ The word cedar comes from the Arabic kedron, meaning "power."

❧ Traditionally cedars were grown in graveyards as they were thought to promote longevity; the wood was used for coffins.

❧ The oil was exported from the Lebanon to ancient Egypt, where the wood was thought to be imperishable, for use in embalming, cosmetics, and perfume.

❧ It is used as a temple incense in modern-day Tibet.

❧ The oil is thought to enhance spirituality and to strengthen the connection with the divine.

❧ It is one of the ingredients of "mithridat," an ancient antidote to poison.

❧ The oil is used as a fragrance and fixative in cosmetic and household products, such as soaps and detergents, as well as in perfumes and men's fragrances.

ABOVE *In Tibet, the people use Atlas cedarwood both in their traditional medicine and as a temple incense.*

HEALTH NOTES

EFFECT ON THE SKIN
• Can be useful for acne, dandruff, dermatitis, dry or combination skin, eczema, greasy skin, skin eruptions, and ulcers.
• Useful for fungal infections such as athlete's foot.
• Has been known to stimulate hair growth and so can be helpful in case of alopecia.

PSYCHOLOGICAL AND EMOTIONAL USES
• Has a calming and soothing effect, and can be a good aid to meditation.
• Has a lingering aroma that can elevate and stimulate the mind and the psyche, and has an invigorating quality that can lift depression, and release anxiety or fear.
• Said to be able to steer you back to the right path.

RIGHT *Use Atlas Cedarwood as a spiritual tool and a meditation aid.*

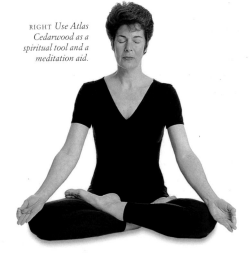

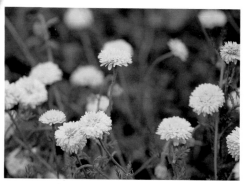

CHAMOMILE OIL

Roman chamomile

CHAMAEMELUM NOBILIS

'he Ancient Egyptians dedicated it to the sun god Ra, and Greek physicians prescribed it for fevers. One of the nine sacred herbs of the Lacnunga, the ancient Anglo-Saxon text, chamomile has been renowned since ancient times for its healing powers.

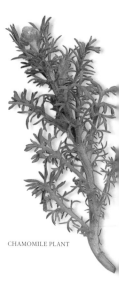

CHAMOMILE PLANT

Distribution
Britain, Germany,
France, Morocco,
Hungary, Belgium,
Italy, U.S.A.

ABOVE *When in full flower, a bed of chamomile fills the senses with a delicious apple-like scent.*

General description
A small perennial herb with feathery, slightly furry leaves and white flowers. The whole plant has a wonderful apple-like aroma.

Attributes and characteristics
Comforting, healing, mild, soothing, tonic, warming. Similar in its action to the more expensive blue chamomile (Matricaria chamomilla).

RIGHT *Daisy-like flowers, feathery pinnate leaves, and a hairy stem characterize this pretty and aromatic plant.*

PROPERTIES

Family name **COMPOSITAE**

Method of extraction
Steam distillation of dried flower heads.

Chemical constituents
Angelic, methacrylic, tiglic (acids); azuline (sesquiterpene). Azuline is not present in the plant but forms in the oil.

Note
Middle.

Aroma
Strong, dry, and fruity.

Properties
Analgesic, antiallergenic, antianemic, anticonvulsive, antidepressant, antiemetic, antineuralgic, antiphylogistic, antipruritic, antirheumatic, antiseptic, antispasmodic, bactericidal, carminative, cholagogue, cicatrisant, digestive, diuretic, emmenagogue, emollient, febrifuge, hepatic, hypnotic, nervine, sedative, splenetic, stomachic, sudorific, tonic, vermifuge, vulnerary.

Blends
Angelica, bergamot, clary sage, geranium, jasmine, lavender, neroli, patchouli, rose, sweet marjoram, ylang-ylang.

USES THROUGH THE AGES

❧ The common name is derived from the Greek expression kamai melon, meaning "ground apple."

❧ The genus name nobilis means "nobility" or "noble."

❧ The ancient Egyptians held it sacred and dedicated it to Ra, their sun god.

❧ It was used in Egypt to treat all fevers and for anointing the body.

❧ It was known as "maythen" to the Saxons and was one of their nine sacred herbs.

❧ It was later dedicated to St. Anne, the mother of the Virgin Mary.

❧ The Elizabethans used it in their homes to get rid of unpleasant odors.

❧ It is traditionally used to lighten hair color, and chamomile tea is known for its ability to aid digestion and restful sleep.

❧ In Tudor times chamomile lawns were popular for their hardiness and the smell they gave off when they were walked on.

❧ It has been known as the "plants' physician" because it cures neighboring plants of their ailments.

RIGHT Worshiped above all other herbs, the ancient Egyptians dedicated chamomile to Ra, the sun god.

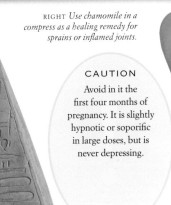

HOME USE

• Alleviates muscular pain, especially if connected to nervous conditions and stress.
• Can be used for arthritis, headaches, neuralgia, toothache, teething pain, and earache.
• Good in compresses for treating sprains and inflamed joint conditions.
• Can regulate the menstrual cycle and ease period pain.
• Relieves premenstrual syndrome and helps any problems associated with the menopause.
• Improves the digestion and soothes the stomach. It can help with irritable bowel syndrome,

diarrhea, colic, vomiting, wind, and bowel inflammation.
• Can alleviate jaundice and liver problems.
• Has an affinity with the genito-urinary system and can help with cystitis.
• Stimulates the production of white blood cells, which fight infection and strengthen the immune system.
• Good for dealing with any emotional or stress-related conditions that manifest themselves physically, including those that appear as skin conditions.

RIGHT Use chamomile in a compress as a healing remedy for sprains or inflamed joints.

HEALTH NOTES

EFFECT ON THE SKIN
• Benefits burns, blisters, inflammations, ulcers, boils, and wounds.
• Can help hypersensitive skin, acne, athlete's foot, herpes, dermatitis, psoriasis, and allergic conditions.
• Good for dry, itchy skin.
• Improves skin elasticity.

PSYCHOLOGICAL AND EMOTIONAL USES
• A very relaxing oil, removing anxiety, tension, anger, and fear.
• Promotes a feeling of ease, comfort, and peace, and allays worries.
• Very beneficial for insomnia.

CAUTION
Avoid in it the first four months of pregnancy. It is slightly hypnotic or soporific in large doses, but is never depressing.

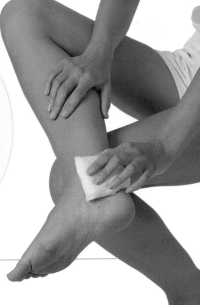

Lime

CITRUS AURANTIFOLIA

*A digestive stimulant, lime is a traditional remedy for indigestion,
heartburn, and nausea. It is used to treat fevers, coughs, colds,
and sore throats and its astringent qualities make it an excellent and
refreshing skin care product.*

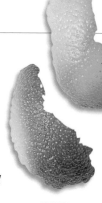

LIME PEEL

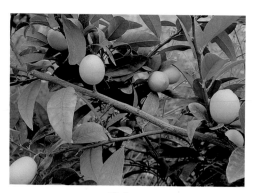

ABOVE *The lime grows on
medium-sized evergreen trees.
The fruit ripens from yellow to
green.*

General description

A small evergreen tree with smooth leaves and small
white flowers. The ripe fruit is green and, on average,
smaller than a lemon.

Attributes and characteristics

Antiseptic, appetite stimulating, cooling, refreshing, tonic.

BELOW *The lime fruit is
bitter tasting and about
half the size of a lemon.*

PROPERTIES

Family name **RUTACEAE**

Method of extraction
*Expression from the unripe
fruit and its peel. A large
quantity of essential oil is
distilled from the whole
fruit, that has a more lime-
like smell.*

Chemical constituents
*Linalool, terpineol
(alcohols); Citral
(aldehyde); linalyl acetate
(ester); bergaptene (lactone
– only found in the
expressed oil, not the
distilled oil); limonene,
pinene, sabinene,
terpinolene (terpenes).*

Note
Top.

Aroma
Light, sweet, and rich.

Properties
*Analgesic, antidepressant,
antimicrobial, antipyretic,
antioxidant,
antirheumatic,
antiscorbutic, antiseptic,
antiviral, aperitif,
astringent, bactericidal,
carminative, deodorant,
disinfectant, febrifuge,
galactagogue, hemostatic,
insecticidal, nervine,
restorative, sedative
(nervous), tonic.*

Blends
*Angelica, bergamot, blue
gum eucalyptus, geranium,
grapefruit, juniper,
lavender, neroli, Roman
chamomile, rose,
sandalwood, sweet fennel,
ylang-ylang.*

CAUTION

The expressed oil may cause
photosensitivity in strong sunlight,
although the distilled oil will not.
Use the oil in moderation as it
may irritate sensitive skin.

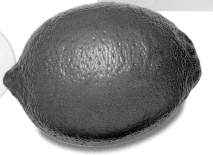

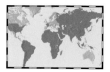

Distribution
Originally from Asia. Now
cultivated in Italy, West Indies,
U.S.A., Mexico.

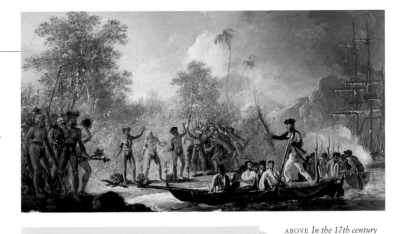

USES THROUGH THE AGES

🌿 It was introduced to Europe by the Moors, and to America by Spanish and Portuguese explorers around the 16th century.

🌿 English ships carrying limes were called "lime juicers" as their crews depended on the fruit to prevent scurvy, a vitamin C deficiency that causes general weakness. The nickname "limey" for British sailors derives from this and is now used to refer to any English person.

🌿 It was once used as a traditional remedy for dyspepsia (indigestion, heartburn, and nausea) with glycerin of pepsin.

🌿 The fruit and juice industry started in the West Indies in the 19th century, and lime is now used to flavor cola and ginger ale.

ABOVE *In the 17th century English sailors ate limes to protect against scurvy.*

HOME USE

• Can help cool fever, especially when this is accompanied by coughs, colds, and sore throats.
• Eases chest congestion, sinusitis, and catarrh.
• As a tonic to the immune system, it brings new energy after an illness.
• As a digestive stimulant, it helps to encourage the secretion of digestive juices.
• Its disinfecting and restorative processes can

alleviate the effects of alcoholism.
• Can be helpful with rheumatic pain and arthritis.
• Can help relieve varicose veins as it encourages good circulation.
• Makes an excellent warming bath in winter and a refreshing, stimulating one in the summer months.

HEALTH NOTES

EFFECT ON THE SKIN
• Astringent, toning, and refreshing, especially to those with greasy skin.
• Can help to stem bleeding from cuts and wounds (use in a compress, not neat on the wound).

PSYCHOLOGICAL AND EMOTIONAL USES
• Very stimulating, especially where there are feelings of apathy, anxiety, and depression.
• Refreshes and uplifts a tired mind.

BELOW *16th-century Portuguese navigators (seen here with astrolabe), introduced limes to the Americas.*

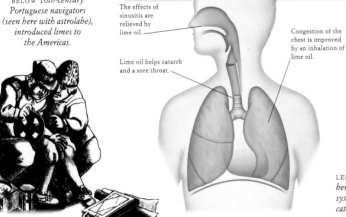

The effects of sinusitis are relieved by lime oil.

Lime oil helps catarrh and a sore throat.

Congestion of the chest is improved by an inhalation of lime oil.

LEFT *Lime is extremely beneficial to the respiratory system, aiding bronchitis, catarrh, and asthma.*

Neroli

CITRUS AURANTIUM

Named after an Italian princess, neroli, or orange blossom, was traditionally used in bridal bouquets to calm a nervous bride. It is a popular ingredient in cosmetics and perfume both for its beautiful smell and positive effect on dry, sensitive, and mature skin.

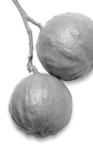

NEROLI FRUIT

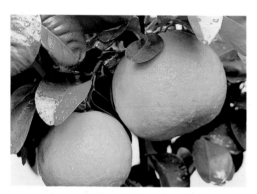

ABOVE *The neroli fruits or bitter oranges are both smaller and darker than those found on the sweet orange tree.*

General description

An evergreen tree with glossy dark green leaves, aromatic white flowers and rich orange fruit. The orange tree produces three essential oils: neroli from the blossom, orange from the fruit, and petitgrain from the leaves and twigs. Petitgrain has similar qualities to neroli but is not as refined. Orange oil has similar qualities to the other citrus oils especially lemon, and mandarin.

Attributes and characteristics

Antidepressant, aphrodisiac, hypnotic, soothing to the nerves (especially in difficult times).

RIGHT *The aromatic white flowers are set against glossy dark green leaves.*

PROPERTIES

Family name **RUTACEAE**

Method of extraction
Steam distillation of orange blossom petals, a flower water and an absolute also result from this process. A concrete and absolute are also produced by solvent extraction, Oil of neroli is also produced by enfleurage.

Chemical constituents
Phenylacetic (acid); nerol, geraniol, linalool, nerolidol, terpineol (alcohols); linalyl acetate, methyl anthranilate, neryl acetate (esters); jasmone (ketone); camphene, limonene (terpenes).

Note
Middle to base.

Aroma
Heady, sweet, and floral with fruity undertones.

Properties
Antidepressant, antiseptic, antispasmodic, aphrodisiac, bactericidal, carminative, cicatrisant, cordial, cytophylactic, deodorant, digestive, emollient, fungicidal, hypnotic (mild), stimulant (nervous), tonic (cardiac, circulatory).

Blends
Bergamot, clary sage, frankincense, geranium, jasmine, lavender, lemon, lime, myrrh, Roman chamomile, rose, rosemary, sandalwood, ylang-ylang.

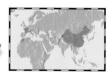

Distribution
France, Morocco, Portugal, Italy. The orange tree originally comes from China.

USES THROUGH THE AGES

Its name derives from Princess Anne Marie of Nerola, in Italy, who loved to wear this oil as a perfume.

The properties of neroli oil were not recognized until the 16th century, although the therapeutic effects of oranges had been acknowledged since at least the 1st century.

In Venice, neroli was acclaimed for its ability to combat plague and fever. It was also drunk as a tea in order to help overcome nervousness.

In China neroli petals were used in making cosmetics. It was also an ingredient (along with bergamot, lemon, lavender, and rosemary) of eau-de-Cologne, used in treating the vapors.

Today the white blossoms are often used in bridal bouquets as a symbol of purity, both for their beauty and for their ability to calm the bride's nerves.

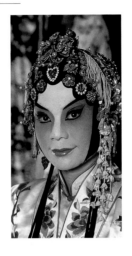

RIGHT *The Chinese used neroli petals to make cosmetics.*

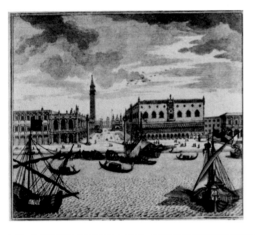

LEFT *Venetians traditionally used neroli as a remedy against plague and fever.*

TIP

It is nontoxic, nonirritant, and nonsensitizing, and is very relaxing indeed.

HOME USE

• A heart regulator, good for palpitations and cleansing the blood.
• Improves circulation.
• Has a positive effect on the sympathetic nervous system, soothing and aiding restful sleep.
• Is an aphrodisiac and calms anxiety.
• Relieves premenstrual discomfort and distress, and helps with the irritability and tearfulness that can accompany the menopause.
• Antispasmodic for the intestines and can improve colon problems, diarrhea, and nervous dyspepsia.
• Eases the pain of neuralgia and headaches.

HEALTH NOTES

EFFECT ON THE SKIN
• Helps regenerate skin cells and improves skin elasticity (dry, sensitive, and mature skins respond best to it).
• Can help with acne, thread veins, scarring, and stretchmarks.

PSYCHOLOGICAL AND EMOTIONAL USES
• Hypnotic and euphoric – a natural tranquilizer.
• Relieves chronic anxiety, depression, and stress, it soothes hysteria, shock, and panic, and it gives a feeling of peace.

• Re-energizes, gives confidence, and lifts mental lethargy.

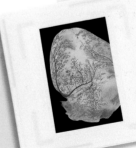

ABOVE *Use neroli to cleanse the blood and regulate the heart.*

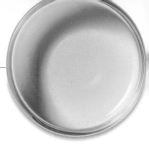

Bergamot

CITRUS BERGAMIA

BERGAMOT OIL

*Traditionally used in Italian folk medicine, bergamot in named for the
Italian city of Bergamo in Lombardy. The essential oil is particularly useful
for the treatment of mouth, skin, respiratory, and urinary tract infections
and may also be used to regulate the appetite.*

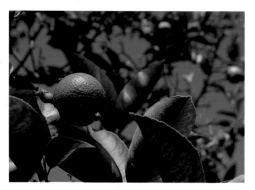

ABOVE *Similar to a miniature
orange in appearance, the bergamot
fruit ripens to yellow.*

PROPERTIES

Family name **RUTACAEA**

Method of extraction
*Cold expression from
fruit peel.*

Chemical constituents
*Linalool, nerol, turpineol
(alcohols); linalyl acetate
(ester); bergaptene
(lactone); dipentene,
limonene (terpenes).*

Note
Top.

Aroma
*Spicy, delicate scent. Light
and refreshing.*

Properties
*Analgesic, antidepressant,
antiseptic, antispasmodic,
carminative, cicatrisant,
cordial, deodorant,
digestive, expectorant,
febrifuge, insecticidal,
sedative, stomachic, tonic,
vermifuge, vulnerary.*

Blends
*Blue gum eucalyptus,
cypress, geranium, juniper,
jasmine, lavender, lemon,
mandarin/tangerine,
neroli, patchouli, Roman
chamomile, sweet
marjoram, ylang-ylang.*

General description

A small tree with long, smooth, oval, green leaves and
white flowers. Bears small, round fruit that ripen from
green to yellow. Should not to be confused with the
decorative herb Monarda didyma, which is also
occasionally called bergamot.

Attributes and characteristics

Antidepressant, antiseptic,
balancing, calming, insect
repellent, refreshing, sedative
(nervous system), uplifting.

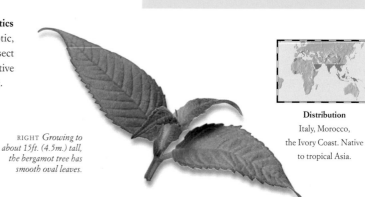

RIGHT *Growing to
about 15ft. (4.5m.) tall,
the bergamot tree has
smooth oval leaves.*

Distribution
Italy, Morocco,
the Ivory Coast. Native
to tropical Asia.

CAUTION

It is advisable to avoid strong sunlight and sunbeds after using this oil on the skin, as it can increase photosensitivity. It is possible to buy bergamot oil that has had the furocoumarins (that can cause the photosensitivity) removed.

EFFECT ON THE SKIN

- Was once used in tanning lotions but it is now known that it can cause dark pigmentation to appear on skin exposed to direct sunlight.
- Can prove beneficial to oily skin conditions, especially if these are stress-related.
- Can help acne, eczema, psoriasis, scabies, varicose ulcers, wounds, herpes, and seborrhea of the skin and scalp.

PSYCHOLOGICAL AND EMOTIONAL USES

- Oil has a soothing effect on the nervous system.
- Aroma has an uplifting effect on the mind.
- A natural balancer, it can help with anxiety, depression, and grief.
- Cool and refreshing, it is enhances the brain's receptivity to light.
- Can prove very beneficial when you are run down and exhausted from constant stress, or if you are convalescing from a psychological or physical illness.

USES THROUGH THE AGES

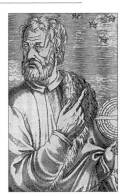

- It is named for Bergamo, the town in Italy where the tree was originally cultivated. Legend has it that Christopher Columbus took the tree from the Canary Islands to Spain and Italy.

- Bergamot is used to flavor Earl Grey tea (efforts at creating this blend in the home are not recommended), and is a common ingredient in eau-de-Cologne.

- In voodoo, bergamot essence is used to protect against evil and danger and to anoint participants in initiation rituals.

ABOVE *Christopher Columbus is thought to have have introduced the bergamot tree to Spain and Italy.*

CAUTION

Bergamot oil may irritate sensitive skin when used in a high concentration, although in moderation it has a positive effect on sensitive skin.

HOME USE

- Has an affinity with the urinary tract, and is helpful for cystitis and other bladder infections, especially when used in combination with Roman chamomile in a compress or mild local wash.
- Can be helpful in the event of painful indigestion, flatulence, hemorrhoids, dyspepsia, and colic.

- Can be an appetite regulator.
- Limits the activity of both the herpes simplex virus that causes cold sores, and the herpes zoster virus that causes chicken pox and shingles.
- Good for respiratory problems such as bronchitis.
- Can be a good insect repellent.

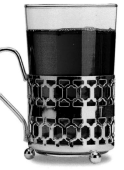

ABOVE *The ever-popular Earl Grey tea is flavored with bergamot which gives it its distinctive flavors.*

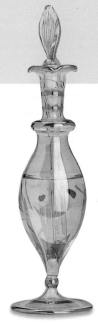

ABOVE *Bergamot is one of the ingredients in eau-de-cologne.*

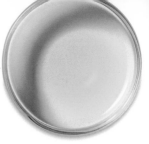

Lemon

CITRUS LIMON

LEMON OIL

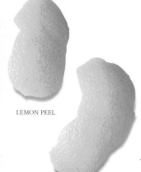

LEMON PEEL

High in vitamins C, the lemon can prove valuable in the cantainment and treatment of infectious diseases, particularly colds and fevers. It is also used extensively as a refreshing fragrance in soaps, cosmetics, and perfumes.

ABOVE *Native to Asia, lemon trees are now cultivated worldwide for their fruits.*

PROPERTIES

Family name **RUTACEAE**

Method of extraction
Expression from the fruit and fruit peel.

Chemical constituents
Linalool (alcohol); citral, citronellal (aldehydes); cadinene (sesquiterpene); bisabolene, camphene, dipentene, limonene, phellandrene, pinene (terpenes).

Note
Top.

Aroma
Bright, fresh, and sharp.

Properties
Antianemic, antimicrobial, antineuralgic, antipruritic, antirheumatic, antisclerotic, antiscorbutic, antiseptic, antitoxic, astringent, bactericidal, carminative, cicatrisant, depurative, diuretic, emollient, escharotic, febrifuge, hemostatic, hepatic, hypoglycemiant, hypotensive, insecticidal, laxative, rubefacient, stimulant, stomachic, tonic, vermifuge.

Blends
Blue gum eucalyptus, frankincense, geranium, ginger, juniper, lavender, neroli, Roman chamomile, rose, sandalwood, sweet fennel, ylang-ylang.

General description

An evergreen tree with shiny leaves, pink and white perfumed flowers, and bright yellow fruit.

Attributes and characteristics

Antiseptic, cephalic, refreshing, strengthening, tonic to the nervous and circulatory systems.

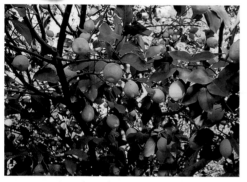

RIGHT *Both lemon peel and juice are widely used as a flavoring agent and as a rich source of vitamins.*

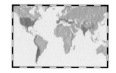

Distribution
Southern Europe, U.S.A., Argentina. Native to India.

USES THROUGH THE AGES

 The Egyptians used lemon oil as an antidote to fish and meat poisoning.

 It was once thought to be valuable in treating malaria and typhoid, and has been used to perfume clothes and repel insects.

 The fruit was carried aboard Royal Navy ships during the 17th century in order to prevent scurvy (vitamin C deficiency) among English sailors.

 Research in Japan has shown that inhaling lemon oil can greatly increase concentration levels.

 It is now used in hospitals for its antiseptic properties and for its ability to neutralize unpleasant odors.

 In medical research it has been found to have a psychologically strengthening effect on patients who are either frightened or depressed.

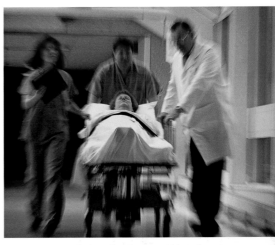

ABOVE *Lemon oil products are widely used in hospitals for their antiseptic and aromatic qualities.*

HOME USE

* A heart and circulatory tonic that can lower the blood pressure.
* Good for relieving the pressure of varicose veins and for arteriosclerosis.
* Stimulates the production of both white and red blood cells, alleviating anemic conditions and boosting the immune system.
* Inhaled, it can help to stop a nosebleed.
* Improves the digestion and makes the contents of the stomach less acidic.
* Helps to clear and stimulate the kidneys and liver.
* Can help with constipation, obesity caused by a congested system, and cellulite.
* Balances acid conditions in the body and helps with ulcers, gout, and arthritis.
* Relieves coughs, colds, and flu conditions, especially when accompanied by fever as it can lower the body temperature.
* A good insect repellent.

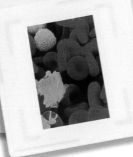

RIGHT *Lemon oil boosts the immune system and stimulates the production of new blood cells.*

HEALTH NOTES

EFFECT ON THE SKIN
* Brightens dull complexions as it helps to remove dead skin cells.
* A mild bleach.
* A good cleanser for greasy skin and hair, and can help with dandruff.
* Can help to soften scar tissue and toughen up fingernails.
* Good for verrucas, corns, and warts. Neat lemon oil can be used directly on the affected area, but it is important not to let it touch the surrounding skin.

PSYCHOLOGICAL AND EMOTIONAL USES
* Can be both refreshing and cooling.
* Clears, refreshes, and stimulates the mind, and is helpful with listlessness and emotional confusion.
* Good for premenstrual syndrome and stress.

CAUTION

It may irritate sensitive skin; in such cases use in very low dosage. It is best to avoid direct sunlight immediately after use since it may have a mild phototoxic effect.

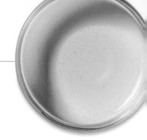

Grapefruit

CITRUS PARADISI

GRAPEFRUIT OIL

In common with other citrus fruits, grapefruit is high in Vitamin C and is often used in the treatment of colds and flu. Its uplifting and reviving qualities make it a popular and effective oil for use at home in a burner to counteract depression or nervous exhaustion.

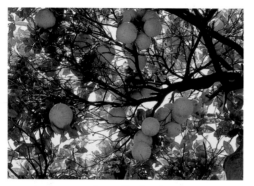

ABOVE *Large yellow fruits hang in abundance from the trees in this cultivated orchard in California.*

General description
A cultivated tree with glossy leaves, white flowers, and large yellow fruit that hang from the tree like massive bunches of grapes.

Attributes and characteristics
Antiseptic, diuretic, cleansing, tonic to the central nervous system and the sympathetic nervous system.

PROPERTIES

Family name RUTACEAE

Method of extraction
Cold expressed from fresh peel. Some oil is distilled from what remains after the expression process but it is of inferior quality.

Chemical constituents
Geraniol, linalool (alcohols); citral (aldehyde); limonene, pinene (terpenes).

Note
Top.

Aroma
Sweet, sharp, and refreshing.

Properties
Antidepressant, antiseptic, antitoxic, aperitif, astringent, bactericidal, depurative, diuretic, disinfectant, resolvent, stimulant (lymphatic, digestive), tonic.

Blends
Atlas cedarwood, bergamot, frankincense, geranium, jasmine, lavender, lemon, neroli, Roman chamomile, rose, rosemary, rosewood, sweet basil, ylang-ylang.

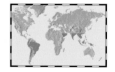

RIGHT *Much of the grapefruit crop is now cultivated in the state of California, U.S.A.*

Distribution
Israel, Brazil, California, Florida. Native to tropical Asia and the West Indies.

HEALTH NOTES

EFFECT ON
THE SKIN

- It can help clear acne and congested or oily skin.
- It promotes hair growth and tones the skin and tissues.

PSYCHOLOGICAL AND
EMOTIONAL USES

- It is uplifting and reviving, and so is valuable in the burner for stress, depression, and nervous exhaustion.

- It can be both euphoric and hypnotic.
- It may have a balancing effect on the central nervous system and has been used to stabilize manic depression.
- It can relieve the discomfort of headaches and be helpful in dealing with performance stress of any sort.

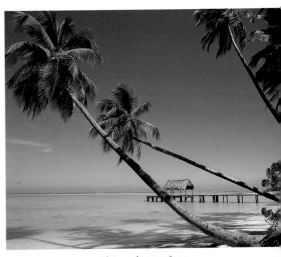

ABOVE *The grapefruit was first cultivated in the West Indies during the 18th century.*

BELOW *Grapefruit oil has a stimulating and uplifting effect.*

TIP

Nontoxic, nonirritant, nonsensitizing, nonphototoxic. Has a short life in the bottle: Keep the top well screwed on.

USES THROUGH
THE AGES

It originated in Asia, although today it is often grown in the Mediterranean.

Legend has it that the fruit was first cultivated in the West Indies during the 18th century, where it was named Shaddock fruit after the captain who transported it there.

The U.S.A. made it big business to grow grapefruit in the 1930s and remains the world's largest producer.

HOME USE

- It is a lymphatic stimulant, and so can nourish tissue cells and control fluid processes.
- It can have a positive effect on obesity and fluid retention, and its diuretic properties may also help to clear cellulite.
- It is good for exercise preparation, and for muscle fatigue and stiffness. It stimulates bile, and so can help fat digestion and possibly weight loss (always use it externally).
- It can be a stimulant to the appetite as it has balancing effect on the digestive system.

- It cleanses the kidney and vascular system, and is a tonic to the liver.
- It can be of benefit in supporting the body during drug withdrawal.
- It is good for jetlag as it can help to minimize headaches and tiredness.
- It has a soothing effect on the body generally, and can alleviate migraine, premenstrual syndrome, and discomfort during pregnancy.
- It can be a support to the immune system in dealing with colds and flu.
- When used in a burner it is particularly effective for purifying the air and killing airborne germs.

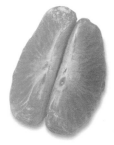

Mandarin/tangerine

CITRUS RETICULATA

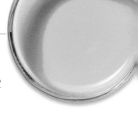

MANDARIN OIL

The mandarin gets its name from the Mandarins of China to whom it was a traditional gift. Nontoxic and non-irritant, this oil is regarded as a safe remedy for children's indigestion. It may also be given to the elderly to strengthen the digestive system.

MANDARIN
SEGMENT

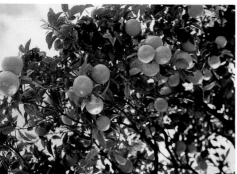

ABOVE *Mandarin and tangerine trees come from the same botanical source and flourish in hot climates.*

General description

Tangerines are from a lower stage of the horticultural development of the fruit, and grow on small evergreen trees with glossy leaves and fragrant flowers. The modern tangerine is more like the original Chinese mandarin fruit, being larger, rounder and having a yellower skin.

Attributes and characteristics

Appetite stimulating, cleansing, balancing, gentle, liver and digestive tonic. Mandarin oil is the safest remedy for children's indigestion. This is also the first oil to try on your child's skin since it is so mild, although you should still always use it well diluted.

RIGHT *The tangerine is seedless, unlike the mandarin.*

PROPERTIES

Family name **RUTACEAE**

Method of extraction
Expressed from peel.

Chemical constituents
Limonene (terpene) and citral (aldehyde) are common to both. Mandarin: geraniol (alcohol); citronellal (aldehyde); methyl anthranilate (ester). Tangerine: citronellol, linalool (alcohols); cadinene (sesquiterpene),

Note
Top.

Aroma
Sweet, light, and tangy. Mandarin oil has floral undertones.

Properties
Antiseptic, antispasmodic, carminative, cholagogue, cytophylactic, digestive, diuretic (mild), emollient, laxative (mild), sedative, stimulant (digestive and lymphatic), tonic.

Blends
Bergamot, grapefruit, lavender, lemon, neroli, Roman chamomile, sweet basil, sweet marjoram, ylang-ylang.

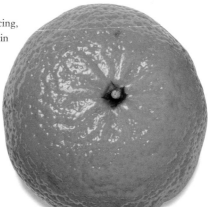

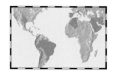

Distribution
Mandarin: Italy, Spain, Algeria, Cyprus, Middle East, Brazil. Tangerine: Texas, Florida, California, Guinea.

USES THROUGH THE AGES

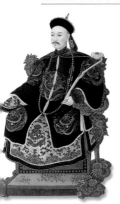

ABOVE *The mandarin gets its name from the Mandarins of China, to whom they were offered as a gift.*

🎋 Chinese officials were called mandarins, and the fruits were named after them because they were traditionally offered as a token of respect.

🎋 The mandarin was brought to Europe in 1805. It arrived in America 40 years later, where it was renamed the tangerine as it was imported from Tangier in Morocco.

🎋 The names mandarin, tangerine, and satsuma are used almost interchangeably, although the oils produced from the fruits are quite different from one another.

TIP
Both mandarin and tangerine are very safe to use in pregnancy. It has been said that mandarin oil is better for the morning and tangerine oil for the evening. Both oils may be mildly phototoxic, although this has not been shown conclusively.

HOME USE

• Both mandarin and tangerine oils encourage appetite, especially after depression.
• Stimulate the liver and regulate the metabolic processes, as well as encouraging the secretion of bile and the breakdown of fats.
• Help with fluid retention and cellulite.
• Calm the intestines.

• Can have a revitalizing and strengthening effect, and can improve peripheral circulation.
• Help with insomnia.
• In a blend of other oils they help to ease premenstrual syndrome.
• Both mandarin and tangerine oils, although mild, have a powerful effect if used in a synergistic combination with other oils.

BELOW *Use a few drops of mandarin or tangerine oil in a bath to aid restful sleep.*

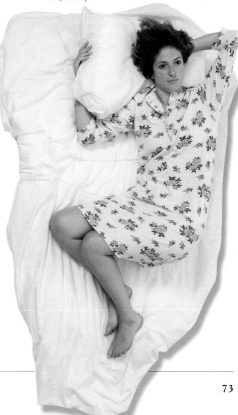

HEALTH NOTES

EFFECT ON THE SKIN
• Both oils lessen stretchmarks and scarring, especially when used in combination with neroli and lavender.
• Can tone the skin and help with the healing of scars and spots, and can also help to clear acne and congested or oily skin.

PSYCHOLOGICAL AND EMOTIONAL USES
• Uplifting and revitalizing, and banish depression and anxiety.
• Good post-illness tonics.
• Tangerine has a hypnotic effect and can calm the central nervous system.

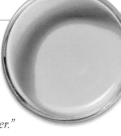

Myrrh

COMMIPHORA MYRRHA

The name derives from the Arabic word "murr," which means "bitter." It has been in use for at least 3,000 years and is recognizable by its powerful scent. It is used to treat asthma, coughs, colds, catarrh, and sore throats. Skin complaints, including ringworm and eczema, may also be treated with myrrh.

MYRRH OIL

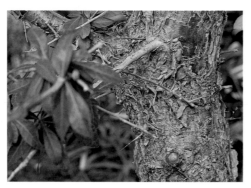

ABOVE *The myrrh tree is native to northeast Africa, India, and the Middle East.*

General description

A shrub or small tree up to 33ft. (10m.) high with knotted branches, aromatic leaves, and small white flowers.

Attributes and characteristics

Healing, purifying, revitalizing, soothing, uplifting.

PROPERTIES

Family name **BURSERACEAE**

Method of extraction
Steam distilled from a natural oleo resin, taken from the trunk, stem, and branches.

Chemical constituents
Myrrholic (acid); cinnamic, cuminic (aldehydes); eugenol (phenol); cadinene (sesquiterpene); dipentene, heerabolene, limonene, pinene (terpenes).

Note
Base.

Aroma
Hot, bitter, and musty.

Properties
Anticatarrhal, anti-inflammatory, antimicrobial, antiphylogistic, antiseptic, astringent, balsamic, carminative, cicatrisant, deodorant, disinfectant, diuretic, emmenagogue, expectorant, fungicidal, stimulant, stomachic, sudorific, tonic, uterine, vulnerary.

Blends
Cypress, frankincense, geranium, juniper, lavender, mandarin/tangerine, patchouli, sandalwood, Scotch pine, tea tree, vetiver.

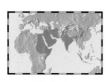

Distribution
Middle East, India, northeast Africa.

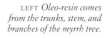

LEFT *Oleo-resin comes from the trunks, stem, and branches of the myrrh tree.*

USES THROUGH THE AGES

 The Vedas and Koran both talk of myrrh being used in religious ceremonies and as a healing agent.

 Myrrh is also mentioned in the Bible. It was a gift from the Magi to the infant Jesus, was present at the Crucifixion, and is referred to in the Song of Solomon.

The Egyptians burned myrrh every day as part of their sun-worshiping rituals. They also used it for treating herpes and hayfever, and stuffed the stomachs of corpses with it in the mummification process.

According to Greek mythology, Myrrha, the daughter of the king of Cyprus, was transformed into a shrub by Aphrodite as a punishment for incest.

Greek soldiers took a phial of myrrh into battle; its antiseptic and anti-inflammatory qualities made it very helpful for cleaning and healing wounds.

In traditional Tibetan medicine it is still employed as a remedy for stress and nervous disorders.

In China it is used for arthritis, menstrual problems, sores, and hemorrhoids.

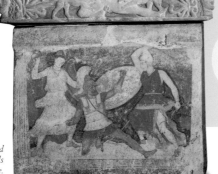

RIGHT *Greek soldiers used myrrh to clean wounds received in battle.*

HEALTH NOTES

EFFECT ON THE SKIN
• Has powerful preservative properties that can be effective in preventing the spread of gangrene.
• Has a cooling action that may alleviate ulcers, sores, wounds, and dry, chapped skin.
• Can help weeping eczema, athlete's foot, and ringworm.

• Can help to rejuvenate mature complexions and smooth out wrinkles.

PSYCHOLOGICAL AND EMOTIONAL USES
• Can lift feelings of weakness, apathy, and lack of incentive.
• Cools heated emotions.
• Like frankincense, it has a gently calming effect on the nervous system and can instill peace and tranquillity of mind.

CAUTION
This oil is best avoided during pregnancy. Do not use in high concentrations.

BELOW *Myrrh is an excellent remedy in the treatment of sore throats or pharyngitis.*

HOME USE

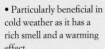

• Particularly beneficial in cold weather as it has a rich smell and a warming effect.
• Can be helpful for rheumatism.
• Known as the "mucus mover" because of its ability to dry out excess fluids.

• Excellent for clearing the respiratory system. It can help with colds, sore throats, catarrh, pharyngitis, and coughs.
• Can be beneficial in cases of glandular fever and also asthma, bronchitis, and voice loss.
• Good for viral infections.

• Can clear obstructions from the womb, help with thrush, and encourage scanty periods.
• Calms and stimulates the digestive system and restores the appetite.
• Stimulates the white blood cells and is a tonic to the immune system.

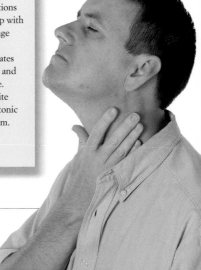

Cypress

CUPRESSUS SEMPERVIRENS

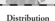

CYPRESS
CONES

*Considered sacred by both the Ancient Egyptians and the Romans, the
cypress is still used as a purifying incense by the Tibetans. It is used to
regulate bodily fluids, particularly diarrhea or heavy menstrual loss.
Its calming qualities make it an appropriate oil to use in times of stress.*

ABOVE *The cypress is a tall
evergreen tree, that now
grows all over Europe .*

PROPERTIES

Family name **CUPRESSACEAE**

Method of extraction
*Steam distillation from
fresh leaves, needles, twigs,
and cones. A small
quantity of absolute and
concrete can also be
produced.*

Chemical constituents
*Sabinol (alcohol); furfurol
(aldehyde); terpenyl
acetate (ester); camphene,
cymene, pinene,
sylvestrene (terpenes).*

Note
Middle to base.

Aroma
*A clear, refreshing, and
tenacious odor.*

Properties
*Antirheumatic, antiseptic,
antispasmodic,
antisudorific, astringent,
cicatrisant, deodorant,
diuretic, febrifuge,
hemostatic, hepatic,
insecticidal, restorative,
sedative, styptic, tonic,
vasoconstrictor.*

Blends
*Bergamot, clary sage,
juniper, lavender, lemon,
mandarin/tangerine,
Roman chamomile,
rosemary, sandalwood,
sweet marjoram.*

General description

A tall, conical-shaped evergreen tree, with hard,
reddish-brown wood and brown/gray cones.

Attributes and characteristics

Antiseptic, comforting, purifying,
refreshing, warming.

RIGHT *The essential
oil is extracted from
the needles, twigs,
and the cones of the
cypress tree.*

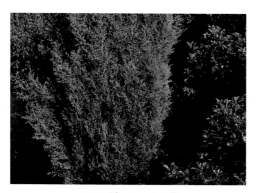

Distribution

Native to the Mediterranean, now
grown all over Europe. Cultivation
and distillation often take place in
Morocco, Spain, and France.

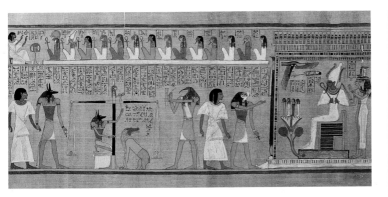

USES THROUGH THE AGES

🌿 There is a legend that Christ's Cross was made from cypress wood.

🌿 The Greeks and Romans grew cypress trees in their burial grounds.

🌿 The Egyptians used the wood for making coffins and for its medicinal properties, and both the Egyptians and Romans dedicated the tree to their gods of death and the underworld.

🌿 Sempervirens means "lives forever," although one of its folk names is "tree of death."

🌿 It is still burned in Tibet as a purification incense.

🌿 In Western magic, ritual objects are purified and consecrated in its smoke.

ABOVE *As a symbol of immortality, the Ancient Egyptians dedicated the cypress to their gods of death.*

CAUTION

It is best not to use it in pregnancy, as it can regulate the menstrual cycle. Take great care if applying it in dilution to varicose veins: never massage directly over or below the veins, as even the gentlest pressure may be detrimental.

HEALTH NOTES

EFFECT ON THE SKIN
• Can be beneficial for a mature skin because it can balance fluid loss.
• Can help to rebalance excessively sweaty or oily skin and aid the healing of wounds.

PSYCHOLOGICAL AND EMOTIONAL USES.
• Overtalkative people benefit most from its calming qualities, and it can have a positive effect on anger.
• Can be helpful in times of transition and stress, such as career change, moving house, bereavement, or the end of a relationship.

HOME USE

• Can help to regulate excess of any kind in the body, particularly fluids.
• Useful for nosebleeds, edema, incontinence, unusually excessive sweating, and heavy, painful menstrual periods.
• May help reduce cellulite and improve poor circulation.

• Has a balancing effect on the female reproductive system and can help with menopausal problems.
• Can be helpful for varicose veins and hemorrhoids.
• A tonic to the circulation and balances excess heat.
• Has an antispasmodic effect on coughs that

accompany flu, on bronchitis, and on whooping cough.
• Particularly useful in a burner for children because of its calming and reassuring properties as well as its respiratory benefits.
• An insect repellent.

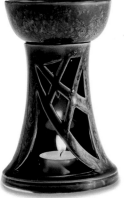

ABOVE *Use cypress oil in a burner to calm restless children or as an aid to the respiratory system.*

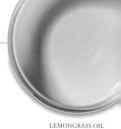

Lemongrass

CYMBOPOGON CITRATUS

LEMONGRASS OIL

Lemongrass is used in traditional Indian medicine in the treatment of infectious diseases and to bring down fever. Both humans and animals benefit from its use as an insect repellent. It is a digestive stimulant and is often used to flavor food.

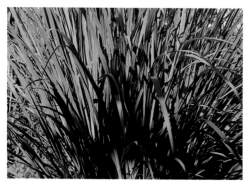

ABOVE *The sturdy pointed leaves of the tropical moisture-loving lemongrass grow to over 6ft. (1.8m.) high.*

General description

A fast-growing, tall, aromatic red grass that quickly exhausts the nutrients in the soil in which it grows.

Attributes and characteristics

Antidepressant, antiseptic, invigorating, stimulating, toning.

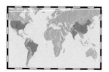

Distribution
India, U.S.A., Brazil,
Sri Lanka, China,
the West Indies.

PROPERTIES

Family name **POACEAE (GRAMINEAE)**

Method of extraction
Steam distillation from finely chopped grass.

Chemical constituents
Farnesol, geraniol, nerol (alcohols); citral, citronellal (aldehydes); limonene, myrcene (terpenes).

Note
Top.

Aroma
Lemony, with rich overtones.

Properties
Analgesic, antidepressant, antimicrobial, antiseptic, antioxidant, antipyretic, astringent, bactericidal, carminative, deodorant, digestive, diuretic, febrifuge, fungicidal, galactagogue, insecticidal, nervine, prophylactic, sedative (nervous), stimulant, tonic.

Blends
Atlas cedarwood, bergamot, blue gum eucalyptus, geranium, ginger, jasmine, lavender, myrrh, neroli, niaouli, patchouli, Roman chamomile, rosemary, sweet basil, tea tree, yarrow.

LEFT *Lemongrass leaves are long, thin, and pointed. They also have a very strong and distinctive fragrance.*

USES THROUGH THE AGES

A favorite oil in traditional Indian medicine, used for bringing down fever, containing infectious diseases, and slowing down the development of tumors.

It is also sometimes known as Indian verbena and Indian melissa oil.

It was also used traditionally to heal skin complaints and kill germs.

Modern Indian research has shown that it has a sedative effect on the central nervous system, and has validated its antiseptic and bactericidal properties.

India was the main supplier until after World War II, when production was taken over by the West Indies.

Exposure to the air and light lowers the citral content of the oil (that makes up 70–85 percent of the oil).

It is a common ingredient in soaps, detergents, perfumes, and cosmetics, and is popular as a food flavoring, particularly in Thai cuisine.

BELOW *Lemongrass is a traditional remedy in Indian medicine.*

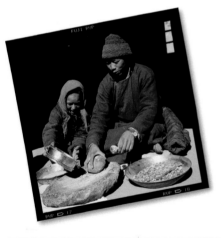

CAUTION

It may irritate sensitive skin: use it in low dosage. An adulterated version of lemongrass is sometimes sold as lemon verbena, although there is also an essential oil of the lemon verbena plant (Lippia citriodora).

HOME USE

• Boosts the parasympathetic nervous system and is a good post-illness tonic.
• Stimulates the appetite and can be beneficial for gastro-enteritis, colitis, and indigestion because it stimulates glandular excretions and the muscles used in digestion.
• Relieves varicose veins and chilblains.
• Its strong antiseptic properties make it beneficial for use in the sickroom, especially for laryngitis, sore throats, fevers, and infectious disease of any kind.

• Eliminates uric acid, adds tone, and improves circulation in tired and aching muscles.
• Can help overcome the hazards of jetlag, overtiredness, and headaches.
• A good insect repellent and deodorant.
• Repels moths.
• Can be used on animals (in dilution) to protect them from fleas and ticks.
• Can aid the flow of breast milk in nursing mothers.

BELOW *Use lemongrass to repel moths.*

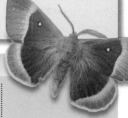

HEALTH NOTES

EFFECT ON THE SKIN
• Tones the skin and may help tighten up loose skin caused by excessive weight loss.

• Can be useful against athlete's foot and other fungal conditions.
• Can balance oily skin conditions and excessive perspiration.

PSYCHOLOGICAL AND EMOTIONAL USES
• Lifts the spirits and gets things moving.
• Is stimulating, reviving, and energizing.

• Can help with nervous exhaustion and any stress-related conditions.

Blue gum eucalyptus

EUCALYPTUS GLOBULUS

A traditional remedy in Australia for respiratory complaints such as bronchitis and croup, blue gum eucalyptus has many healing properties. It is particularly effective in the treatment of burns, blisters, and insect bites. Also used to treat tropical diseases such as malaria, typhoid, and cholera.

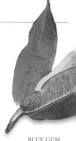

BLUE GUM
EUCALYPTUS LEAF

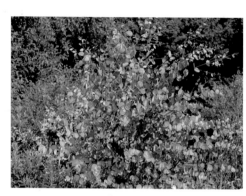

ABOVE *When mature, the blue gum eucalyptus trees produce attractive creamy-white flowers.*

PROPERTIES

Family name **MYRTACEAE**

Method of extraction
Steam distillation of the fresh or partly dried leaves and twigs of the blue gum tree.

Chemical constituents
Citronellal (aldehyde); cineole (ketone); camphene, fenchene, phellandrene, pinene (terpenes).

Note
Top.

Aroma
Clean, sharp, and piercing. It has a distinctive camphoraceous aroma with a sweet undertone that can clear the head.

Properties
Analgesic, antineuralgic, antiphlogistic, antirheumatic, antiseptic, antispasmodic, antiviral, bactericidal, balsamic, cicatrisant, decongestant, deodorant, depurative, diuretic, expectorant, febrifuge, hypoglycemiant, insecticidal, parasiticidal, prophylactic, rubefacient, stimulant, vermifuge, vulnerary.

Blends
Bergamot, juniper, lavender, lemon, lemongrass, melissa/lemon balm, rosemary, Scotch pine.

General description

An attractive tall, evergreen tree with bluish-green, oval leaves, or long, narrow, yellowish leaves in an older tree. It has creamy-white flowers and gray bark that is often covered in a white powder.

Attributes and characteristics

Antiseptic, antiviral, cooling, pain relieving. It can often effectively clear the head.

RIGHT *Blue gum eucalyptus oil is extracted from the leaves and twigs of the tree by steam distillation.*

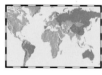

Distribution
Australia and now also Spain, Brazil, California, Russia, China.

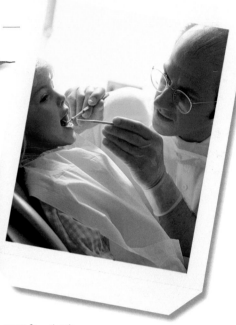

EFFECT ON THE SKIN
• Can be helpful in treating burns and skin conditions, including herpes.
• Its antiseptic and antibacterial qualities can help limit infection.
• Clears congested skin.

PSYCHOLOGICAL AND EMOTIONAL USES
• Can cool down the emotions and clear the head, and can also aid concentration.

• Can be burned to clear the air after an argument.
• Strengthens the nervous system and has a stimulating effect.

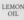

LEMON OIL

JUNIPER OIL

ABOVE *Its antiseptic properties make it ideal for use in dentistry products.*

RIGHT *Blend blue gum eucalyptus with juniper and lemon oils as a remedy for rheumatoid arthritis.*

USES THROUGH THE AGES

Australian Aborigines crush the leaves and apply them to the skin to heal wounds, fight infection, and relieve muscular pain.

A solution of eucalyptus has been used by Western surgeons to wash out operation cavities.

In India it is used to cool fever and contain contagious disease.

It is used in many pharmaceutical products, especially vapor rubs and other cold and chest products, as well as in veterinary medicine and dentistry.

BELOW *The native people of Australia use blue gum eucalyptus to help heal wounds and fight infection.*

CAUTION
Do not use it if you have high blood pressure or epilepsy. Always use it in dilution. It can be a skin irritant if used in large quantities. May be an antidote to homeopathic remedies.

HOME USE

• Good for any respiratory problems because of its decongestant properties.
• Can clear the head of stuffiness in the case of colds or hayfever.
• A good antiseptic and has antiviral properties.
• Can be effective in disinfecting a room, especially in the case of infectious or contagious disease.
• Useful for insect bites, burns, wounds, and blisters, and is also helpful for chilblains.

• Has an affinity with the genito-urinary system and can help with both cystitis and diarrhea.
• Can alleviate rheumatism, including rheumatoid arthritis and fibrositis, especially if used in combination with juniper and lemon oils.
• An insect repellent, especially if used in combination with bergamot and lavender essential oils.
• Can remove tar from clothes or skin (always apply it in dilution).

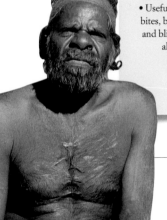

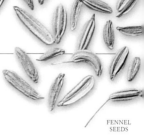

Sweet fennel

FOENICULUM VULGARE

FENNEL
SEEDS

Thought to offer protection against evil, fennel was one of the nine sacred herbs of the Anglo-Saxons. Romans soldiers ate fennel to promote good health and their ladies ate it to prevent obesity. In the 9th century the emperor Charlemagne declared it to be an essential plant for every imperial garden.

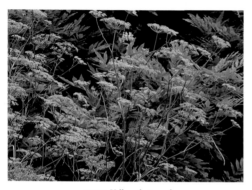

ABOVE *Yellow clusters of flowers and feathery leaves characterize fennel.*

PROPERTIES

Family name UMBELLIFERAE

Method of extraction
Steam distilled from crushed seeds.

Chemical constituents
Anisic, cuminic (aldehydes); fenchone (ketone); anethone, methylchavicol (phenols); camphene, dipentene, limonene, phellandrene (terpenes).

Note
Top to middle.

Aroma
Distinctively aniseedy, spicy, and peppery.

Properties
Anti-inflammatory, antimicrobial, antiphylogistic, antiseptic, antispasmodic, aperitif, carminative, depurative, detoxicant, diuretic, emmenagogue, expectorant, galactagogue, insecticidal, laxative, resolvent, splenetic, stimulant (circulatory), stomachic, sudorific, tonic, vermifuge.

Blends
Geranium, lavender, lemon, rose, rosemary, sandalwood, sweet basil.

General description

Foeniculum vulgare has green, feathery leaves, golden-yellow flowers, and oblong-shaped fruits. There are two varieties of fennel: bitter or common fennel, and sweet or garden fennel. Sweet fennel has a gentler nature and contains less fenchone.

Attributes and characteristics

Balancing, cleansing, insect repellent, revitalizing, stimulating.

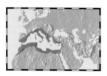

Distribution
Originally Mediterranean, now cultivated extensively worldwide.

LEFT *Growing up to 6ft. (2m.) high, sweet fennel has aromatic lime-green feathery leaves.*

USES THROUGH THE AGES

It was popular with the ancient Chinese and Hindus, who both used it as an antidote to snakebites.

The Egyptians, Chinese, Indians, and Greeks all used it to achieve long life, courage, power, and strength.

The Greeks named the herb marathron, from maraino, meaning "to grow thin."

BELOW *It is used in Asia to neutralize poisons, including snake bites.*

Greek athletes chewed fennel seeds to gain stamina and strength, and Roman gladiators added it to their food for the same reasons.

In medieval England it was known as fenkle, and was thought to to able to ward off evil spirits.

It is traditionally used to strengthen the eyesight and is a basic ingredient of children's gripewater.

In pharmaceutical preparations it is called codex.

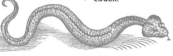

HEALTH NOTES

EFFECT ON THE SKIN
• Has a cleansing and tonic action, especially on dull, oily, or wrinkly skin.
• Can help to heal bruising and slow bleeding.

PSYCHOLOGICAL AND EMOTIONAL USES
• Encourages strength and courage, and is good for self-esteem.
• Calms the nervous system.
• Said to ward off the ill thoughts of others.

CAUTION

Fennel oil is perfectly safe when used in moderation. However, avoid if you are pregnant or epileptic. It is also best not to use it on young children. In very large doses it can have a narcotic effect.

HOME USE

• An excellent detoxifying body cleanser after overindulgence in food or alcohol.
• A good tonic for the digestive system, liver, kidneys, and spleen.
• Can ease indigestion, flatulence, and diarrhea, especially when they are stress-related.
• May help with weight loss because of its natural estrogen content. This can help to balance the metabolism, but can also be a stimulant to the appetite (always use it externally).
• Good for irregular periods and menopausal problems, again because of its natural estrogen content. It can also help with menstrual cramps, premenstrual syndrome, and exhaustion, especially when brought on by too much physical activity.
• Can help to stimulate the flow of breast milk.
• Can relive hiccups, nausea, and vomiting.
• As a diuretic it can be helpful in reducing cellulite and water retention.
• Both antispasmodic and expectorant, so if inhaled it can be useful for colds and coughs as well as asthma and bronchitis.
• Can be used to clean poison from insect bites.

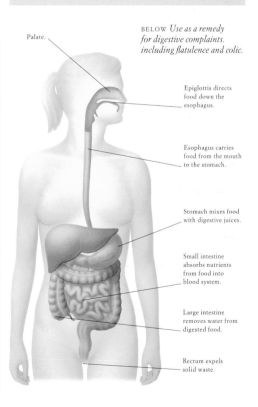

Palate.

BELOW *Use as a remedy for digestive complaints. including flatulence and colic.*

Epiglottis directs food down the esophagus.

Esophagus carries food from the mouth to the stomach.

Stomach mixes food with digestive juices.

Small intestine absorbs nutrients from food into blood system.

Large intestine removes water from digested food.

Rectum expels solid waste.

Jasmine

JASMINUM OFFICINALE

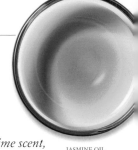

Known in India as "queen of the night" for its rich night time scent, jasmine is used extensively in soaps, cosmetics, and perfumes. In the West it was traditionally used to ease childbirth, while in the East the flowers are used to treat hepatitis and liver cirrhosis.

JASMINE OIL

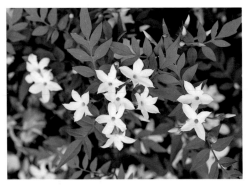

ABOVE *The star-shaped white jasmine flowers provide a wonderful fragrance in any garden.*

PROPERTIES

Family name **OLEACEAE**

Method of extraction
Solvent extraction (formerly enfleurage) from flowers can produce both a concrete and an absolute. Essential oil is produced from the absolute by steam distillation. The extraction process is very delicate and huge quantities of petals are needed to produce the oil.

Chemical constituents
Benzyl, farnesol, geraniol, nerol, terpineol (alcohols); lynalyl acetate, methyl anthranilate (esters); jasmone (ketone); eugenol (phenol).

Note
Base.

Aroma
Sweet, exotic, enduring, and floral.

Properties
Analgesic (mild), antidepressant, anti-inflammatory, Antiseptic, antispasmodic, aphrodisiac, carminative, cicatrisant, emollient, expectorant, galactagogue, parturient, sedative, tonic (uterine).

Blends
Bergamot, clary sage, frankincense, geranium, lime, mandarin/tangerine, melissa/lemon balm, neroli, rose, rosewood, sandalwood, ylang-ylang.

General description

A sturdy, climbing, ever-green shrub with bright green leaves that can grow to a height of 20ft. (6m.). It pro-duces beautifully scented, white, star-shaped flowers that are picked only at night.

Attributes and characteristics

Antidepressant, aphrodisiac, confidence-boosting, intoxicating, reassuring.

RIGHT *The scent of jasmine flowers is even more powerful after nightfall.*

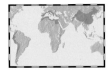

Distribution
Egypt, Morocco, the Mediterranean. Native to Peru, Kashmir, China.

HOME USE

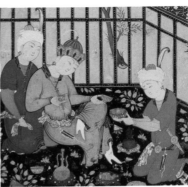

ABOVE *Jasmine oil may provide pain relief during childbirth as well as combat any postnatal blues.*

• Can simultaneously strengthen contractions in childbirth and relieve pain.
• As a hormone balancer it is good for postnatal depression.
• Can relieve menstrual pain and be helpful for any vaginal infection.
• Reputed to increase spermatozoa and can help with both impotence and frigidity – possibly thanks to its relaxing and confidence-inspiring properties.
• Regulates the respiration, deepens breathing, calms spasms of the bronchi, and brings relief to lingering coughs and voice loss.
• Can be beneficial for muscular spasm and sprains.

HEALTH NOTES

EFFECT ON THE SKIN
• A luxurious (expensive, but worth it) tonic. It is excellent for all skin types, particularly for hot, dry, and sensitive skin.
• Applied in a blend with lavender and mandarin/tangerine (and carrier oil) it can encourage cell growth and increase skin elasticity. Use only tiny amounts as overuse can have the opposite effect.

PSYCHOLOGICAL AND EMOTIONAL USES
• Excellent for depression.
• Calms the nerves and warms the emotions by being gentle yet deeply penetrating on an emotional level, especially when employed in massage.
• Can restore confidence, optimism, energy, and vitality.
• Like geranium, jasmine oil can be stimulating or sedative according to individual need.

CAUTION
Do not use in pregnancy until labor is well advanced. At this point it can be very beneficial as it strengthens uterine contractions and relieves pain.

BELOW *Jasmine tea is a popular drink in China.*

RIGHT *Add mandarin, lavender, and jasmine oils to a carrier, such as soya oil, to promote cell growth.*

USES THROUGH THE AGES

Jasmine oil has long been regarded for its aphrodisiac powers.

It is widely used in India for ceremonial purposes.

The Chinese used jasmine to cleanse the atmosphere that surrounded the sick. They also gave it to inebriated guests to clear their heads.

It was used for nervous disorders, including insomnia and headaches.

In China jasmine tea is frequently drunk, and in Indonesia jasmine is used as a garnish to food.

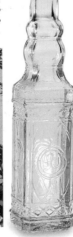

Juniper

JUNIPERUS COMMUNIS

JUNIPER
OIL

JUNIPER
BERRIES

As well as giving gin its characteristic flavor, juniper berries are used extensively in many food products. It has diuretic properties and is good for cystitis and prostate problems. May be used for gastro-intestinal infections and worms. Also helps prevent ticks and fleas.

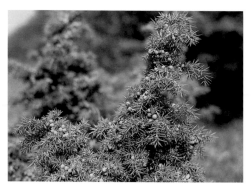

ABOVE *Juniper is a slow-growing coniferous shrub with bluish-green, narrow, stiff needles.*

General description

Has a reddish stem, needle-like leaves, small yellow flowers, and blue berries that turn black on ripening.

Attributes and characteristics

Aphrodisiac, astringent, cleansing, detoxifying, protective, purifying.

Distribution

Hungary, Italy, France, Canada. Native to northern Europe.

PROPERTIES

Family name **CUPRESSACEAE**

Method of extraction
Steam distillation from berries, needles, and wood. A resinoid and concrete are produced in small quantities.

Chemical constituents
Borneol, terpineol (alcohols); cadinene, cedrene (sesquiterpenes); camphene, mercene, pinene, sabinene (terpenes).

Note
Middle.

Aroma
Peppery, clear, and fresh.

Properties
Abortifacient, antirheumatic, antiseptic, antispasmodic, antitoxic, aphrodisiac, astringent, carminative, cicatrisant, depurative, detoxicant, disinfectant, diuretic, emmenagogue, insecticidal, nervine, parasiticidal, parturient, rubefacient, sedative, stimulant, stomachic, sudorific, tonic, vulnerary.

Blends
Bergamot, clary sage, cypress, frankincense, geranium, grapefruit, lavender, lemongrass, lime, melissa/lemon balm, rosemary, sandalwood, vetiver.

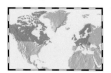

LEFT *The juniper species has spiny needles that bear yellow flowers. The small round berries take up to three years to ripen.*

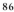

HOME USE

- Relieves fluid retention and the symptoms of cystitis, and eases the flow of urine if the prostate gland is enlarged.
- Can help clear cellulite.
- Regulates the menstrual cycle and can help with cramps and painful periods.
- Detoxifies the liver, intestines, and bladder, especially after too much rich food or alcohol. Also regulates the appetite.
- When used in the bath, it may help combat drowsiness.

- Can clear mucus from the intestines and may help with hemorrhoids. Able to eliminate uric acid, it is beneficial for arthritis, gout, and sciatica.
- Can relieve chilblains.
- Makes a good household disinfectant when diluted with water.

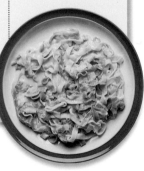

RIGHT *Juniper oil prevents the build up of toxins after too much rich food.*

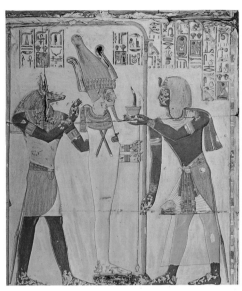

ABOVE *The Ancient Egyptians used juniper oil to anoint corpses before embalming.*

HEALTH NOTES

EFFECT ON THE SKIN
- A tonic for oily and congested skin.
- Good for wet eczema and acne, blocked pores, lice, ticks, fleas, dermatitis, and swellings.

PSYCHOLOGICAL AND EMOTIONAL USES
- Clears, stimulates, and strengthens the mind.
- Known for its ability to support the spirit in challenging situations.
- Good for self-esteem.

CAUTION

Avoid during pregnancy as can induce labor. Best avoided if you have kidney disease as prolonged use may overstimulate the kidneys. Can irritate the skin in large quantities.

USES THROUGH THE AGES

This is one of the earliest aromatics used in ancient civilization; remains of it have been found in a prehistoric dwelling.

The ancient Egyptians used juniper oil to anoint corpses, and used the berries in cosmetics and perfumes and to cure headaches.

In ancient Greece, and also more recently in French hospitals (particularly during the smallpox outbreak of 1870), branches of juniper were burned to combat epidemics.

In England, juniper was burned to scare away witches and demons, and was also used to combat cholera and typhoid fever.

It was considered to be an effective remedy for headaches and capable of restoring lost youth.

The Celtic word juneprus means "acidic" or "biting."

In central Europe the oil was regarded as a miracle cure for typhoid, cholera, dysentery, and tapeworms.

In Mongolia it was given to women at the onset of labor. It is still used as a purification incense in Tibet, and Native Americans burn a form of juniper in their cleansing ceremonies.

The berries are used to flavor gin.

87

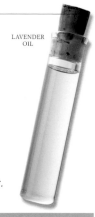

LAVENDER
OIL

Lavender

LAVANDULA AUGUSTIFOLIA

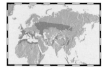

LAVENDER
LEAVES

The dried flower heads were carried by many people during the plague years to ward off the disease. Lavender sachets are still commonly used to scent clothes' drawers and stored bedlinen. The plant's insect repellent qualities will help keep away moths.

ABOVE *Lavender has highly-scented violet-blue flowers in the summer.*

General description

An evergreen shrub with pale green leaves and violet flowers.

Attributes and characteristics

Antidepressant, antiseptic, balancing, calming, cephalic, relaxing.

Distribution

Mediterranean, southern states of former U.S.S.R., Bulgaria, the former Yugoslavia, England, France.

PROPERTIES

Family name **LABIATAE**

Method of extraction
Steam distillation from fresh flowering tops. An absolute and concrete are also produced by solvent extraction.

Chemical constituents
Borneol, geraniol, lavendulol, linalool (alcohols); geranyl acetate, lavandulyl acetate, linalyl acetate (esters); cineole (ketone); caryophyllene (sesquiterpene); limonene, pinene (terpenes).

Note
Middle.

Aroma
Light and floral with clear woody undertones.

Properties
Analgesic, anticonvulsive, antidepressant, antimicrobial, antiphlogistic, antirheumatic, antiseptic, antispasmodic, antitoxic, antiviral, bactericidal, carminative, cholagogue, choleric, cicatrisant, cordial, cytophylactic, decongestant, deodorant, detoxicant, diuretic, emmenagogue, fungicidal, hypotensive, insecticidal, nervine, parasiticidal, restorative, rubefacient, sedative, splenetic, stimulant, sudorific, tonic, vermifuge, vulnerary.

Blends
Bergamot, clary sage, geranium, jasmine, lemon, mandarin/tangerine, neroli, patchouli, Roman chamomile, rose, rosemary, Scotch pine.

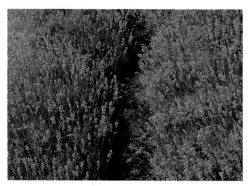

LEFT *The leaves of the lavender plant are narrow and extremely fragrant.*

HEALTH NOTES

EFFECT ON THE SKIN

• Promotes cell growth and balances sebum production, especially in combination with bergamot.
• Accelerates the healing of domestic burns and sunburn.
• Helps to clear acne, athlete's foot, dandruff, eczema, and psoriasis.
• Helpful in healing abscesses, boils, and carbuncles, and in minimizing fungal growths, swellings, scarring, and stretchmarks.
• A tonic to hair growth and is helpful in cases of alopecia.

RIGHT *Lavender has a long lasting fragrance and is one of the oldest and most popular English perfumes.*

PSYCHOLOGICAL AND EMOTIONAL USES

• Helpful to those who suffer from mood swings and feelings of instability.
• Has a balancing effect on the central nervous system and can be helpful in cases of manic depression.
• Soothes the spirit and relieves anger and exhaustion.

CAUTION

If you have low blood pressure you may find lavender makes you slightly drowsy.

USES THROUGH THE AGES

In northern Europe lavender was one of the herbs dedicated to Hecate, goddess of the underworld, and it was said to ward off the evil eye.

Hildegarde von Bingen recommended it in her 12th century herbal for maintaining a pure character.

Lavender is one of the oldest English perfumes and folk remedies, used for its calming, tonic, and insect-repellent properties.

In Elizabethan times women would sew pockets of lavender into their dresses, and even today schoolchildren make lavender bags for clothes drawers.

BELOW *A favorite addition to bathwater, lavender's name derives from the Latin lavare "to wash."*

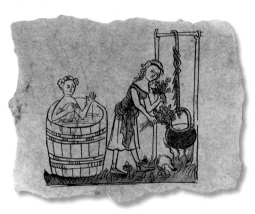

HOME USE

• The most useful oil in therapeutic terms, being sedative, antiseptic, painkilling, and calming.
• Contains many chemicals and has many properties, the most important being to restore balance to all systems of the body.
• Can aid restful sleep and ease headaches.

• Relieves bronchial problems, hayfever, catarrh, flu symptoms, and asthma.
• When blended with sweet marjoram it relieves pain, including muscular sprains, rheumatism, and painful menstrual periods.

• Like jasmine it may be helpful in childbirth, but is best avoided in the early months of pregnancy.
• Can be helpful for nausea, vomiting, and flatulence.
• Stimulates the production of bile and aids the digestion of fats.

• Can lower the blood pressure and prevent palpitations.
• Helps alleviate fluid retention and can relieve the discomfort of cystitis.
• A good insect repellent, and can also be dabbed directly on to stings, bites, wounds, and bruises.

Tea tree

MELALEUCA ALTERNIFOLIA

*The curative properties of the oil distilled from the twigs and spiky leaves
of this Australian tree are truly impressive, making it the focus of considerable
medical research. It has long been respected by the aboriginal people
of Australia, who use it to treat infected wounds.*

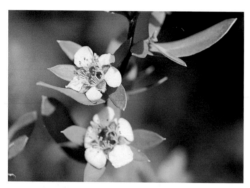

ABOVE *Tea tree is a small tree
or shrub, native to Australia,
mainly New South Wales.*

PROPERTIES

Family name **MYRTACEAE**

Method of extraction
*Steam distillation from
leaves and twigs.*

Chemical constituents
*Terpineol (alcohol); cineole
(ketone); cymene, pinene,
terpinene (terpenes).*

Note
Top.

Aroma
Warm, fresh, and clean.

Properties
*Antibiotic, anti-
inflammatory, antipruritic,
antiseptic, antiviral,
bactericidal, balsamic,
cicatrisant, cordial,
expectorant, fungicidal,
insecticidal, parasiticidal,
stimulant (immune
system), sudorific,
vulnerary.*

Blends
*Blue gum eucalyptus, clary
sage, cypress, ginger,
lavender, lemon,
mandarin/tangerine,
rosemary, thyme, Scotch
pine, ylang-ylang.*

General description

A tree or shrub with needle-like leaves
and yellow or purplish flowers. In the
wild it thrives in marshy areas, but it is
now grown in plantations.

Attributes and characteristics

Antifungal, antiviral, and antibacterial.

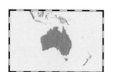

Distribution
Australia.

LEFT *Tea tree oil is
distilled from both
the leaves and twigs
of the plant.*

HEALTH NOTES

EFFECT ON THE SKIN
• Cleansing and antiseptic.
• Can clear blemishes left by chicken pox and shingles, and is good for cracked and rough skin.
• Good for acne, burns, blisters, chilblains, cold sores, warts, athlete's foot, sunburn, herpes, insect bites, varicose veins, and dandruff. It can be dabbed directly onto problem spots (avoid the surrounding area) or used with water in a compress, local wash, or hair rinse. Be careful not to massage directly over or below a varicose vein.

PSYCHOLOGICAL AND EMOTIONAL USES
• Can be refreshing and revitalizing, especially after a shock.

CAUTION

It can be used neat in a first-aid application, but it is best to carry out a patch test first. Limit usage to the problem area, avoiding the surrounding skin.

USES THROUGH THE AGES

🌿 It has been long acknowledged by the Australian Aborigines, who use it to treat infected wounds.

🌿 It was named by Captain Cook's crew, who brewed a drink from its leaves, and was introduced to Europe around 1927, where it was quickly recognized for its antiseptic and germicidal properties.

🌿 During World War II it was included in first-aid kits carried by soldiers fighting in tropical areas and kept in munitions factories as a treatment for skin injuries.

🌿 The oil is a relatively new addition to aromatherapy, although it was soon recognized as an immunostimulant.

🌿 Research has been carried out in France, U.S.A., and Australia on its anti-infectious and antiviral powers, particularly in relation to skin conditions.

BELOW *Second World War soldiers stationed in the tropics used tea tree oil to treat wounds.*

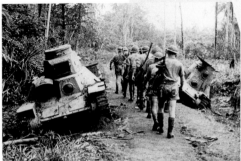

HOME USE

• The use of tea tree oil encourages a very powerful resistance to infection and strengthens the immune system.
• Good in cases of flu and catarrh.
• Has an affinity with the respiratory system and can help with whooping cough, tuberculosis, asthma, bronchitis, and sinusitis.
• Can help the body throw off repeated infections and debilitating illnesses such as glandular fever.
• It is being tested for its efficacy against AIDS.
• Helps to relieve thrush, caused by the fungus *Candida albicans*.
• Relieves itching and the symptoms of cystitis.
• Protects against scarring during deep breast radiotherapy: the oil creates a protective layer on the skin.

• Massage with tea tree in a carrier oil can help to prepare the body before an operation. It can also help to relieve postoperative shock, although it is important to avoid massaging over the operation wound or scar.
• Good for middle ear infections and intestinal inflammation, and can evict intestinal parasites.

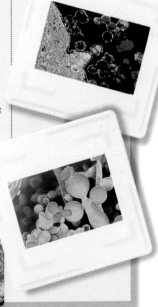

ABOVE TOP *Tea tree is being tested for use against the AIDS virus.*

ABOVE *Relieves thrush, caused by the fungus* Candida albicans.

Niaouli

MELALEUCA VIRIDIFLORA

*Native to Australia and New Caledonia, niaouli is used locally to treat a wide
range of ailments. Its strong antiseptic properties make it ideal for use in hospitals.
It is also used in pharmaceutical products such as gargles, toothpastes, and mouth
sprays, and is sometimes used to purify water.*

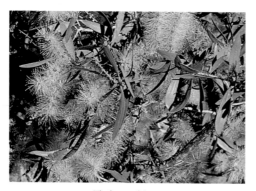

ABOVE *The leaves of the evergreen
niaouli plant are extremely
aromatic when they are crushed.*

PROPERTIES

Family name MYRTACEAE

Method of extraction
*Steam distilled from fresh
twigs, leaves, and shoots.
The irritant aldehydes are
often removed.*

Chemical constituents
*Valeric (acid); terpineol
(alcohol); cineole (ketone);
limonene, pinene
(terpenes).*

Note
Top.

Aroma
*Sharp, clear, and
penetrating.*

Properties
*Analgesic, anticatarrhal,
antirheumatic, antiseptic,
antispasmodic,
bactericidal, balsamic,
cicatrisant, decongestant,
expectorant, febrifuge,
insecticidal, regulator,
stimulant, vermifuge,
vulnerary.*

Blends
*Juniper, lavender, lemon,
lime, myrtle, rosemary,
Scotch pine, sweet fennel.*

General description

An evergreen tree with pointed
leaves and spiky yellow flowers.

Attributes and characteristics

Antiseptic, clearing and cleansing,
physical and mental stimulant.

RIGHT *The niaouli oil is
distilled from the fresh leaves
and young twigs of this tree.*

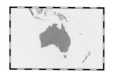

Distribution
New Caledonia, Australia.

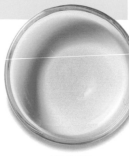

NIAOULI OIL

HOME USE

- A tissue stimulant, particularly of lung tissue, so is good for emphysema, bronchitis, and asthma.
- Stimulates local circulation and increases white blood cell activity.
- A generally healing and stimulating oil, helpful for colds, fevers, and flu.
- Good to use at the beginning of an illness because of its fortifying nature, and it is also useful when you are in a weakened condition.
- Clearing for the respiratory tract, ear, nose, and throat.
- Beneficial for catarrh, laryngitis, bronchitis, flu, whooping cough, and tuberculosis.
- Good for intestinal and urinary infections, including internal parasites.
- Can help to relieve the pain of muscle tension, rheumatism, and neuralgia.
- Used medically in radiation therapy for cancer: a thin layer of niaouli oil is applied to the skin before each session to protect it against burning.
- The tissue-stimulant properties of the oil encourage burns to heal more quickly.

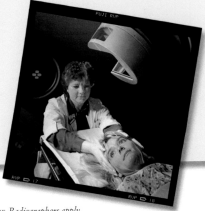

ABOVE *Radiographers apply niaouli oil to the skin to prevent burning during radiation treatment.*

CAUTION

Nontoxic, nonirritant, nonsensitizing. It can often be adulterated and occasionally confused with (or blended with) cajaput oil, which has similar properties but is a skin irritant. Be sure to buy only good-quality niaouli oil. As it is a powerful stimulant, use it late in the evening only in combination with more sedative oils.

BELOW RIGHT *Niaouli has found a place in the Middle Eastern tea drinking ritual.*

HEALTH NOTES

EFFECT ON THE SKIN
- Because it is nonirritant, powerfully antiseptic, and firms the tissues, it may be helpful for skin eruptions such as acne, boils, ulcers, cuts, and insect bites.
- A powerful tissue stimulant and will help to heal mild domestic burns.
- Useful in dilution for washing infected wounds.

PSYCHOLOGICAL AND EMOTIONAL USES
- Has a clearing and reviving action on the mind.
- Aids concentration.

USES THROUGH THE AGES

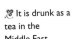

- The healthy air and absence of malaria in New Caledonia is attributed to the niaouli tree.
- It is used in New Caledonia to purify water.
- It is drunk as a tea in the Middle East.
- It was assigned its botanical (Latin) name during Captain Cook's visit to Australia in 1788.
- It has been used in French hospitals in the fields of obstetrics and gynecology for its strong antiseptic properties.

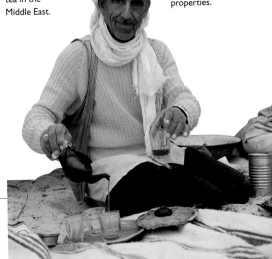

Melissa/lemon balm

MELISSA OFFICINALIS

Used by the Ancient Greeks over 2,000 years ago, melissa was sacred to the goddess Diana. Herbalists have extolled its abilities to banish melancholy for centuries and aromatherapists use it today to relieve depression. It is also used as a fragrance in cosmetics and perfumes.

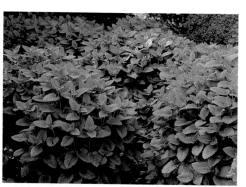

ABOVE *The flavor of melissa leaves is best just as the flowers begin to open. They can be used in salads.*

General description
Sweet-scented herb with bright green serrated leaves and yellow, white, or pink flowers.

Attributes and characteristics
Calming, comforting, soothing, strengthening, uplifting.

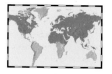

Distribution
Europe, Asia, North America, North Africa, Siberia.

PROPERTIES

Family name **LABIATAE**

Method of extraction
Steam distillation from leaves and flowering tops. All parts of the plant yield essential oil.

Chemical constituents
Citronellic (acid); citronellol, geraniol, linalool (alcohols); citral, citronellal (aldehydes); geranyl acetate (ester); caryophyllene (sesquiterpene).

Note
Middle.

Aroma
Sweet and tangy with floral overtones.

Properties
Antiallergenic, antidepressant, antihistamine, antispasmodic, bactericidal, carminative, choleretic, cordial, digestive, emmenagogue, febrifuge, hypotensive, nervine, sedative, stimulant, stomachic, sudorific, tonic, uterine, vermifuge.

Blends
Frankincense, geranium, ginger, jasmine, juniper, lavender, neroli, Roman chamomile, rose, rosemary, sweet basil, sweet marjoram, ylang-ylang.

MELISSA OIL

LEFT *The bright green serrated leaves of melissa have a strong lemony scent.*

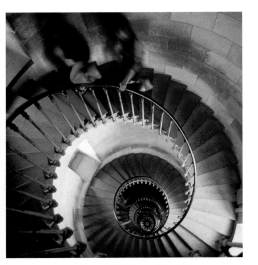

ABOVE *If you suffer from vertigo, melissa oil may help to relieve the symptoms.*

HOME USE

• Regulates menstruation, soothes period pain, and is a tonic to the uterus.
• Calms the heart and lowers the blood pressure, and is useful in cases of fatigue and overstimulation.
• Calms breathing and settles nervous digestion, and is good for indigestion and nausea.

• Can help with colds and chronic coughs, and also cools fevers and soothes migraines and headaches.
• Its antihistamine properties make it good for allergies, including asthma as it can help with breathing difficulties.
• An insect repellent, although it is attractive to bees.

HEALTH NOTES

EFFECT ON THE SKIN
• Can be helpful in cases of greasy hair and baldness.
• Can check the flow of blood in wounds.
• May help to clear fungal infections and eczema.
• Soothes bee stings and insect bites.

CAUTION
As it helps to balance the menstrual cycle it is best avoided in pregnancy. It may irritate sensitive skin, especially as it is frequently adulterated.

PSYCHOLOGICAL AND EMOTIONAL USES
• Can calm those in a state of shock, panic, or hysteria.
• Traditionally, it is known as a tonic for the heart and as a remedy for a distressed spirit.
• Relieves depression, insomnia, and nervous anxiety.
• Balancing on the emotions.
• Helpful for loss and bereavement, including miscarriage, and possibly in preparation for your own death.
• Removes mental blocks and calms hysteria.
• Can help with vertigo.

USES THROUGH THE AGES

Melittena is the Greek word for bee, and Melissa is the name of the Greek nymph who is the insect's protector.

In Greek mythology bees fed honey to the infant Jupiter; melissa honey is reputed to be delicious.

It has been famed for its rejuvenating qualities.

The alchemist Paracelsus called it "the elixir of life."

The plant has long been used therapeutically. It was introduced to Britain in the 4th century by the Romans and has been popular ever since that time.

In Elizabethan times the leaves were used in wine making, and they have also been used as an ingredient in floor polish.

A 16th-century Oxford don recommended it for his students to help clear the head, increase the understanding, and sharpen the memory.

It is often adulterated or blended with cheaper lemongrass or lemon oils as pure melissa is very expensive.

LEFT *The juice of the melissa plant may be added to furniture or floor polish.*

MYRTLE LEAF

Myrtle

MYRTUS COMMUNIS

*Sacred to Venus and the Egyptian goddess Hathor, myrtle is a symbol
of love and purity. Lovers wear it for good luck and happiness and it is often
included in bridal bouquets and headdresses. In Roman times, myrtle was
used as a decoration at weddings and other celebrations.*

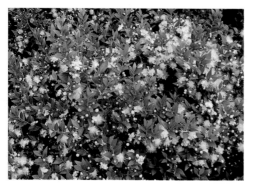

ABOVE *The white blooms of the
myrtle shrub are sweetly scented and
appear from midsummer to autumn.*

General description

A large bush or small tree with many thin
branches, a reddish bark, and small, pointed
leaves. It has white flowers and black berries.
Both leaves and flowers are aromatic.

Attributes and characteristics

Antiseptic, aphrodisiac, refreshing,
stimulating, uplifting.

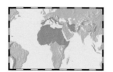

Distribution
Mediterranean,
North Africa, Iran.

PROPERTIES

Family name **MYRTACEAE**

Method of extraction
*Steam distillation from
leaves, twigs, and flowers.*

Chemical constituents
*Geraniol, linalool,
myrtenol, nerol (alcohols);
myrtenal (aldehyde);
cineole (ketone);
camphene, dipentene,
pinene (terpenes).*

Note
Middle.

Aroma
Fresh and penetrating.

Properties
*Anticatarrhal, antiseptic,
astringent, bactericidal,
balsamic, carminative,
expectorant, parasiticidal,
sedative (mild).*

Blends
*Bergamot, clary sage,
ginger, lavender, lemon,
lemongrass, lime, neroli,
rosemary, rosewood,
tea tree.*

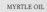

MYRTLE OIL

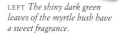

LEFT *The shiny dark green
leaves of the myrtle bush have
a sweet fragrance.*

USES THROUGH THE AGES

The Romans used myrtle for respiratory and urinary problems.

The Egyptians used it for nervous afflictions and steeped the leaves in olive oil to anoint the body.

The Greeks thought of it as a symbol of immortality and used it in love potions.

The winners at the Olympic games were crowned with wreaths of myrtle.

In legend, the goddess Aphrodite sought shelter under a myrtle tree when she emerged from the sea. Since then it has been associated with chaste and pure love.

Some women in the south of France still drink myrtle tea to preserve their looks. It is also traditional to plant a myrtle bush by your door for protection against the evil eye.

In biblical times Jewish women would wear garlands of myrtle to bring good luck.

The leaves and flowers were a major ingredient of the popular 16th-century skin lotion "Angel's Water." At this time, myrtle was thought to cure skin cancers.

More recently, it has become popular in wedding bouquets and headdresses. It is also an ingredient in baby talcum powder.

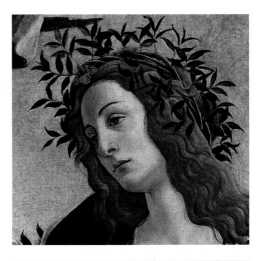

CAUTION
With prolonged use it may irritate mucus membranes.

ABOVE RIGHT *Jewish women wore garlands of myrtle to bring good luck. It is now commonly worn in bridal headdresses.*

HEALTH NOTES

EFFECT ON THE SKIN
• Its antiseptic and astringent qualities mean that it has a cleansing effect on the skin; it can be particularly helpful for oily skin.
• Can be helpful for acne, bruises, and congested skin, especially in washes and compresses.
• May improve the appearance of psoriasis.

PSYCHOLOGICAL AND EMOTIONAL USES
• Has a soothing effect on feelings of anger. It is light, pure, and refreshing and can lift the mood.

HOME USE

• Promotes restful sleep and helps to reduce excessive moisture, including congested lungs, bronchitis, catarrh, and night sweats.
• Can be beneficial to burn myrtle oil in a child's sickroom, particularly at night. It can be massaged into the chest in a very mild dilution with carrier oil or lotion, both as a curative and a preventative measure against respiratory complaints. The smell is not as strong as eucalyptus.
• Has a regulating effect on the genito-urinary system. It can ease diarrhea, hemorrhoids, dysentery, and cystitis and it can be a tonic to the womb.

BELOW *Burn myrtle to relieve congested chests and catarrh. It is also suitable to use for children's coughs.*

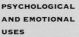

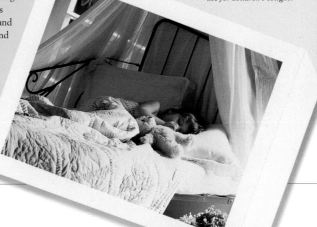

Sweet basil

OCIMUM BASILICUM

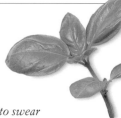

BASIL LEAVES

Basil is considered sacred in Indian culture and it was used to swear oaths upon in court. Legend says that it was found growing around Christ's tomb after the resurrection and Greek Orthodox churches still use it to prepare holy water.

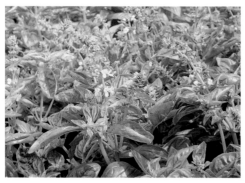

ABOVE *Clusters of small pinkish-white flowers appear on the basil plant in late summer.*

PROPERTIES

Family name **LABIATAE**

Method of extraction
Steam distillation of the whole plant.

Chemical constituents
Linalool (alcohol); borneone, camphor, cineole, (ketones); methylchavicol, eugenol (phenols); ocimene, pinene, sylvestrene (terpenes).

Note
Top.

Aroma
A light, fresh, sweet-spicy scent. The whole plant exhibits a powerful aroma.

Properties
Analgesic, antiallergenic, antidepressant, antiseptic, antispasmodic, antivenomous, aphrodisiac, bactericidal, carminative, cephalic, digestive, emmenagogue, expectorant, febrifuge, galactagogue, insecticidal, nervine, prophylactic, restorative, stimulant, stomachic, sudorific, tonic, vermifuge.

Blends
Bergamot, clary sage, geranium, lavender, lime, melissa/lemon balm, neroli, sandalwood.

General description

An annual herb with dark, hairy, oval leaves and an erect stem that bears pale pink flowers.

Attributes and characteristics

Aphrodisiac, cephalic, clearing, strengthening, insect repellent, uplifting, warming.

SWEET BASIL OIL

LEFT *Basil is a culinary herb with a distinctive and strong aromatic scent.*

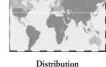

Distribution
North Africa, France, Seychelles, Cyprus, Réunion, U.S.A., South America. Originated in Asia, Africa, Pacific Islands.

CAUTION

Basil is generally a tonic and stimulating oil, but in excess it can have the opposite effect. Avoid during pregnancy.

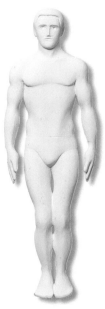

ABOVE *Use sweet basil oil as a remedy for tired and aching muscles.*

HOME USE

• Can be good for headaches, migraines, and chest infections.
• Can help with respiratory allergies such as hayfever and asthma since it has an effect on the adrenal cortex, which controls all stress-related allergies.
• Soothes nausea and digestive problems or upsets, and helps relieve hiccups.
• A good kidney and intestinal cleaner.
• Can imitate natural estrogen and can therefore help to regulate periods.

• Can be beneficial against wasp and insect bites and acts as an insect repellent.
• Can help to lower the body's level of uric acid and so it can also be helpful in cases of gout and arthritis.
• Stimulates blood flow, so it can be beneficial for deep muscle injuries and in bringing new vigor to tired, overworked muscles.

CAUTION

Use basil oil with care as it can irritate the skin. Do not use it neat on the skin; if you know you have sensitive skin dilute it well before use and carry out a patch test before adding to the bathwater.

USES THROUGH THE AGES

Basilikos is Greek for "royal," and it is believed the plant may have been used in an oil for anointing kings.

Indian folklore holds basil sacred to Krishna and Vishnu. Members of the Brahman caste regard basil as a sacred plant capable of giving spiritual and physical protection to anyone who wears it. Its leaves are placed on the breasts of the dead as protection for their soul.

It is much used in Ayurvedic medicine for its antiseptic properties.

In China it is used for stomach and kidney ailments.

It has been regarded as an aphrodisiac for centuries and is a popular culinary herb.

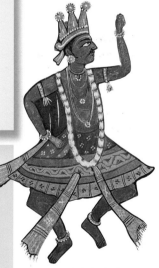

ABOVE *In India, basil is believed to contain a divine essence and is held sacred to the god Krishna.*

HEALTH NOTES

EFFECT ON THE SKIN
• Has a refreshing, cleansing, and tonic action.
• Can benefit congested skin and possibly acne.

PSYCHOLOGICAL AND EMOTIONAL USES
• Has a reviving, refreshing effect on the mind and spirits, and sharpens the senses and the concentration.

• Can help to calm hysteria and balance nervous disorders.
• Can be uplifting if you are depressed.
• Good for those in need of protection after a debilitating illness.

Sweet marjoram

ORIGANUM MAJORANA

Legend says that Aphrodite regarded this sweet smelling herb as a symbol of happiness. In Greece newly married couples were crowned with garlands of marjoram to bring them good fortune. Introduced into Europe in the Middle Ages, marjoram soon became a favorite ingredient of nosegays and bathwaters.

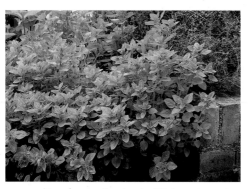

ABOVE *Growing up to 35in. (90cm.) high, sweet marjoram is a hardy bushy perennial herb.*

General description

A perennial herb with dark green, oval leaves and small white flowers. The whole plant has an aroma.

Attributes and characteristics

One of the most sedating, calming, and warming oils, especially for the elderly.

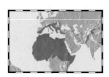

Distribution
Egypt, Morocco, Tunisia, Bulgaria, Hungary. Native to the Mediterranean, Egypt, North Africa.

PROPERTIES

Family name **LABIATAE**

Method of extraction
Steam distilled from dried flowering heads and leaves.

Chemical constituents
Borneol, terpineol (alcohols); camphor (ketone); caryophyllene (sesquiterpene); pinene, sabinene, terpinene (terpenes).

Note
Middle.

Aroma
Warm, heavy, and penetrating.

Properties
Analgesic, anaphrodisiac, antioxidant, antiseptic, antispasmodic, antiviral, bactericidal, carminative, cephalic, cordial, digestive, diuretic, emmenagogue, expectorant, fungicidal, hypotensive, laxative, nervine, restorative, sedative, stomachic, tonic, vasodilator, vulnerary.

Blends
Atlas cedarwood, bergamot, cypress, lavender, mandarin/tangerine, Roman chamomile, rosemary, rosewood, ylang-ylang.

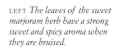

LEFT *The leaves of the sweet marjoram herb have a strong sweet and spicy aroma when they are bruised.*

CAUTION

Marjoram is perfectly safe for home use in dilution. Excessive use may cause drowsiness. It is best avoided during pregnancy and is not suitable for small children

HEALTH NOTES

EFFECT ON THE SKIN
• Good for bruises, chilblains, and ticks, and can improve the circulation.
• Has a comforting and warming effect.

PSYCHOLOGICAL AND EMOTIONAL USES
• Has a calming effect on the central nervous system.

• Relieves anxiety, stress, and possibly deeper emotional trauma, but if overused it can have a deadening effect on the mind.
• Strengthens the mind to confront issues.
• Slows down hyperactivity.

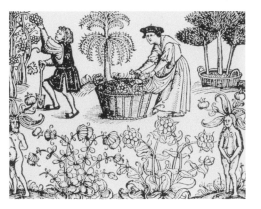

HOME USE

• Powerful in relieving painful muscles and joints.
• Good for menstrual and digestive pain and helps to regulate the menstrual cycle.
• Can clear the body of toxins and may be beneficial in case of seasickness.
• Dilates the arteries and capillaries and improves the circulation, especially to the extremities.

• A tonic to the heart, it can lower blood pressure.
• Helps to clear mucus from the chest and relieves the symptoms of asthma, bronchitis, and sinusitis.
• Good for migraines and insomnia.

USES THROUGH THE AGES

✿ A very popular medicinal herb in ancient Greece, used to calm muscle spasm and relieve excess fluid in the tissues, and also as an antidote to poison.

✿ The Greeks called the herb orosganos, meaning "joy of the mountain," and made garlands of it for newlyweds as a token of good fortune.

✿ It was planted in graveyards and on graves to bring peace to the souls of the departed.

✿ The plant was considered sacred to Osiris in Egypt, and to Vishnu and Shiva in India.

✿ In England sweet marjoram was grown from the 13th century by monks in their herbariums.

✿ The herb was used for nervous complaints and was hung in dairies to stop milk turning sour.

✿ In Stuart Britain sweet marjoram nosegays were carried to hide any unpleasant smells.

✿ It was used in aromatic waters and snuff. Fresh leaves were added to the bath, and the oil was used for insomnia, nausea, and headaches.

✿ It has been employed by religious institutions for its anaphrodisiac properties.

RIGHT *Sweet marjoram was traditionally added to snuff.*

ABOVE LEFT *Sweet marjoram was introduced to England in the Middle Ages and grown by monks in their gardens.*

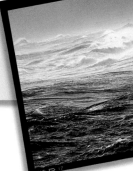

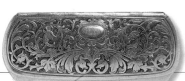

ABOVE *Try using sweet marjoram oil if you suffer from seasickness.*

Geranium

PELARGONIUM GRAVEOLENS

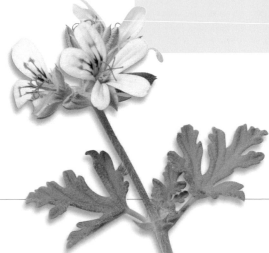

GERANIUM LEAVES

Widely cultivated, the geranium is grown for ornamental use as well as for use in the cosmetic and food industries. It has been used as a remedy for dysentery, cholera, and fractures. Women may find it particularly beneficial for menstrual tension and also during the menopause.

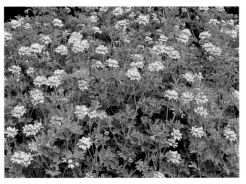

ABOVE *There are over 700 species of geranium but* Pelargonium graveolens *is most commonly planted for its oil.*

General description

Grows to about 2ft. (60cm.) high, and has serrated, pointed leaves and pink, red, or white flowers. The whole plant is scented.

Attributes and characteristics

Balancing, cheerful, tonic, invigorating, uplifting.

PROPERTIES

Family name **GERANIACEAE**

Method of extraction
Steam distillation from leaves, stalks, and flowers. An absolute and concrete can also be produced.

Chemical constituents
Geranic (acid); geraniol, citronellol, linalool, myrtenol, terpineol (alcohols); citral (aldehyde); methone (ketone); eugenol (phenol); sabinene (terpene).

Note
Middle.

Aroma
Sweet, yet penetrating.

Properties
Analgesic, anticoagulant, antidepressant, antihemorrhagic, anti-inflammatory, antiseptic, astringent, cicatrisant, cytophylactic, deodorant, diuretic, fungicidal, hemostatic, hypoglycemiant, insecticidal, styptic, tonic, vasoconstrictor, vermifuge, vulnerary.

Blends
Angelica, Atlas cedarwood, bergamot, clary sage, grapefruit, jasmine, juniper, lavender, lime, mandarin/tangerine, neroli, patchouli, Roman chamomile, rose, rosemary, sandalwood, sweet basil.

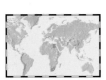

Distribution
Native to South Africa, now cultivated worldwide but the most oil is produced in Réunion and Egypt.

LEFT *Both the green serrated leaves and the small flowers are highly aromatic.*

RIGHT *Geraniums were traditionally planted around a house to prevent evil spirits harming the owners.*

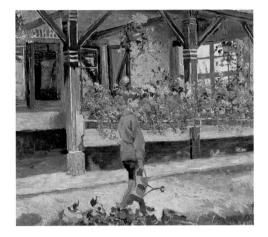

CAUTION

Geranium is perfectly safe in the home if used in moderation. In very great quantities it may cause irritation to sensitive skins.

USES THROUGH THE AGES

❧ Belief in geranium's powers has traditionally led people to plant it around their houses to keep away evil spirits. The herb Robert, a native British species from the same family, was widely used for this purpose before the geranium was imported.

❧ It has variously been respected as a remedy for wounds, tumors, cholera, dysentery, and fractures.

HOME USE

• Has a balancing effect, particularly on the body's hormone levels.
• Has a stimulating effect on the adrenal cortex of the brain, which secretes chemicals to regulate the release of hormones throughout the body.
• Can be useful for premenstrual syndrome and heavy periods, as well as any problems experienced with the menopause.
• Can help to reduce water retention and edema, and is doubly beneficial in treating cellulite as it is also a stimulant to the body's immune system.
• Can have a positive effect on the respiratory system, and can help relieve sore throats and tonsillitis.
• A tonic to both the liver and kidneys, and can help them clear the body of toxins. It can also clear digestive mucus and be a source of support in breaking an addiction.
• A tonic to the circulatory system, making it more fluid.
• Has both a tonic and sedative effect on the nervous system: in a hot bath it is deeply relaxing; in a cooler one it is more energizing.
• Can help relieve headaches.
• A good insect repellent.

HEALTH NOTES

EFFECT ON THE SKIN
• Can prove useful for all types of skin as it balances sebum, the fatty substance that keeps skin supple.
• A good overall skin cleanser and can invigorate a pale skin by improving its circulation. It can also help against acne, dandruff, eczema, burns, shingles, herpes, ringworm, chilblains, and athlete's foot.
• A single drop can be applied directly to a trouble spot.

PSYCHOLOGICAL AND EMOTIONAL USES
• A tonic to the nervous system and so can lift depression (especially if used in combination with bergamot) and reduce stress and nervous tension.

BELOW *May be applied to the foot as a remedy for athlete's foot.*

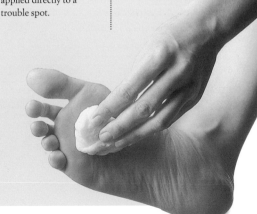

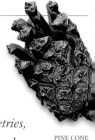

Scotch pine

PINUS SYLVESTRIS

Its distinctive and fresh scent make pine a common component of toiletries, particularly bath products. Used in inhalations to relieve asthma, catarrh, and blocked sinuses. Its restorative properties help combat fatigue and may aid recovery after a long illness.

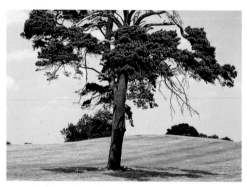

ABOVE *The Scotch pine can grow up to 131ft. (40m.) high.*

General description

A tall evergreen tree with a reddish bark, gray/green needles, pointed brown cones, and orange flowers.

Attributes and characteristics

Antiseptic, comforting, evocative, inspiring, stimulating.

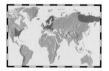

Distribution

Northern Europe, northeast Russia, eastern U.S.A., Scandinavia.

PROPERTIES

Family name **PINACEAE**

Method of extraction
Steam distillation from needles, cones, and twigs.

Chemical constituents
Borneol (alcohol); bornyl acetate, terpinyl acetate (esters); cadinene (sesquiterpene); camphene, dipentene, phellandrene, pinene, sylvestrene (terpenes).

Note
Middle.

Aroma
Sharp, fresh, and clean.

Properties
Antimicrobial, antineuralgic, antiphylogistic, antirheumatic, antiscorbutic, antiseptic (pulmonary, urinary, hepatic), antiviral, bactericidal, balsamic, cholagogue, choloretic, decongestant, deodorant, diuretic, expectorant, hypertensive, insecticidal, restorative, rubefacient, stimulant (adrenal cortex, circulatory, nervous), sudorific, tonic, vermifuge.

Blends
Atlas cedarwood, blue gum eucalyptus, cypress, lavender, myrtle, niaouli, rosemary, tea tree.

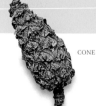

CONE

LEFT *Scotch pine oil is distilled from the needles, pines, and twigs of this large evergreen tree.*

USES THROUGH THE AGES

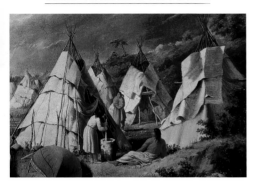

ABOVE *The Native Americans made a drink from pine needles that helped prevent scurvy (Vitamin C deficiency).*

🌿 It was associated with religious ceremonies in ancient Greece, Egypt, and Arabia, and was used for pulmonary conditions such as bronchitis, tuberculosis, and pneumonia, and also for aching muscles.

🌿 Pine needles were burned to clear away infections and insects.

🌿 The ancient Romans ate pine kernels in bread as a restorative.

🌿 Pine-needle mattresses are still used as a remedy for rheumatism in the Swiss Alps.

🌿 The Native Americans brewed the needles as a drink to prevent scurvy and used them as mattress stuffing to repel lice and fleas. The twigs were mixed with cedar and juniper for use as a purification incense.

🌿 Pine branches are used in saunas in Scandinavia.

🌿 Pine oil is often used in bath oils and foams (always in a carrier) for its fresh scent and antirheumatic and neuralgic properties.

CAUTION

It is best to refrain from using Scotch pine oil on sensitive skin and on the skin of children and the elderly. Also avoid this oil if you have high blood pressure as it is a mild hypertensive.

CAUTION

Other pine oils can be toxic, so always use the botanical name to make sure that you buy the right oil. Definitely avoid Pinus pumilio (dwarf pine).

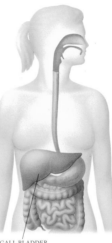

GALL BLADDER

ABOVE *The oil reduces inflammation of the gall bladder and the incidence of gallstones.*

HEALTH NOTES

EFFECT ON THE SKIN
• Can help clear congested skins and have a positive effect on eczema and psoriasis.
• Can be effective for athlete's foot, cuts, skin irritations, scabies, and sores.

PSYCHOLOGICAL AND EMOTIONAL USES
• Refreshes a tired mind.
• Good for feelings of weakness and self-doubt.
• Can alleviate fatigue, nervous exhaustion, and neuralgia.
• The aroma of pine conjures up visions of endless forests and hence imbues a sense of freedom.

HOME USE

• A powerful antiseptic.
• Helpful for chest complaints.
• Eases breathlessness and clears the sinuses.
• Cleanses the kidneys and so can be effective for cystitis, hepatitis, and prostate problems.

• Can act as a stimulant to the adrenal glands and so revitalize the body.
• Warming or cooling depending on the body's needs.
• Can reduce profuse sweating and stimulate the circulation.

• Its warming properties can relieve rheumatism, sciatica, and arthritis.
• Can help with digestive problems.
• Has an affinity for both the male and female reproductive systems.

Patchouli

POGOSTEMON CABLIN

*Native to tropical Asia, patchouli is extensively cultivated
for its oil. In the East it is used to prevent the spread of disease
due to its antimicrobal, antiseptic, and antiviral properties. The herb
is also used as an antidote to poisonous snake bites.*

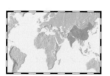

PATCHOULI LEAF

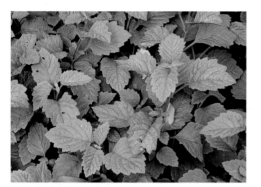

ABOVE *The patchouli has a
powerful musky, spicy, and
oriental scent.*

General description

A bush with furry leaves and purplish white flowers that
quickly drains the nutrients from the soil in which it
grows.

Attributes and characteristics

Antiseptic, aphrodisiac, deodorant, tonic to the nervous system,
uplifting.

PROPERTIES

Family name LAMIACEAE (LABIATAE)

Method of extraction
*Steam distillation from
dried, fermented leaves. A
resinoid that is also
produced is mainly used as
a fixative.*

Chemical constituents
*Patchoulol (alcohol);
benzoic, cinnamic
(aldehydes); eugenol
(phenol); cadinene
(sesquiterpene).*

Note
Base.

Aroma
*Rich earthy, spicy, and
lingering. It improves with
age.*

Properties
*Antidepressant, antiemetic,
anti-inflammatory,
antimicrobial,
antiphlogistic, antiseptic,
antitoxic, antiviral,
aphrodisiac, astringent,
carminative, cicatrisant,
cytophylactic, deodorant,
diuretic, febrifuge,
fungicidal, insecticidal,
nervine, prophylactic,
sedative, stimulant
(nervous), stomachic, tonic.*

Blends
*Atlas cedarwood,
bergamot, clary sage,
frankincense, geranium,
ginger, lavender,
lemongrass, myrrh, neroli,
rose, rosewood,
sandalwood, Scotch pine,
vetiver.*

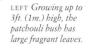

Distribution
India, the Philippines,
China, Malaysia, Paraguay.

LEFT *Growing up to
3ft. (1m.) high, the
patchouli bush has
large fragrant leaves.*

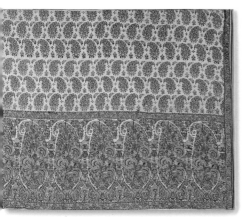

ABOVE *Patchouli was introduced to Britain in the 1820s with the import of Indian fabrics.*

RIGHT *In the 1960s patchouli oil was in great demand as a body perfume.*

USES THROUGH THE AGES

The word patchouli originates in Hindustan. The oil has long been used medicinally in Malaysia, India, China, and Japan for nausea, headaches, colds, vomiting, diarrhea, abdominal pain, and halitosis.

Its antiseptic and antimicrobal properties can prevent the spread of disease and infection.

It is renowned as an antidote to insect and snake bites.

Patchouli first became known in Britain in the 1820s when imported Indian fabrics became fashionable.

Paisley shawls were scented with patchouli to make them more exotic.

Since the 19th century patchouli leaves have been folded into clothes and linen to protect them from moths.

CAUTION

Patchouli is sedative in smaller amounts but stimulating in larger amounts. It may cause loss of appetite. Its challengingly powerful aromas may have a variety of associations. As with other oils, avoid its use if you find the smell unpleasant.

HOME USE

• Has a diminishing effect on the appetite and is therefore good for weight loss (use externally only).

• Tightens up loose skin, especially after rapid or excessive weight loss.

• Thanks to its binding qualities it relieves diarrhea.

• A diuretic, so it can be helpful for cellulite and water retention.

• A natural antiperspirant and deodorant.

• Has a balancing effect on the libido, which is probably related to the balancing effect it has on the endocrine system.

HEALTH NOTES

EFFECT ON THE SKIN
• Can cool inflamed conditions and help heal cracked and dry skin, sores, and wounds.
• Can also help with acne, weeping eczema, athlete's foot, fungal infections, psoriasis, and problems with the scalp such as dandruff.
• Can improve the condition of oily hair and skin.

• Its skin-regenerative properties can help the formation of scar tissue, and its qualities of tissue regeneration encourage the replacement of skin cells.

PSYCHOLOGICAL AND EMOTIONAL USES
• Both grounding and balancing.

• Strengthens and stimulates the nervous system if used in moderation, but is sedative if used excessively.
• Increases clarity and objectivity.
• Useful for depression, frigidity, anxiety, and all stress-related conditions.

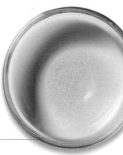

ROSE PETALS

Rose

ROSA CENTIFOLIA OR ROSA DAMASCENA

*Remains of roses have been found in Egyptian tombs, and a red
rose is depicted at the 4,000 year old palace at Knossos in Crete. It was
possibly the first plant matter distilled by Avicenna in his alchemical experiments.
The rose continues to be a symbol of love and purity.*

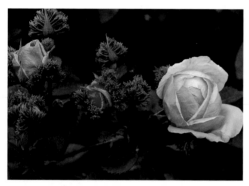

ABOVE *Rose essential oil is
extracted from the beautifully
scented fresh petals.*

General description

Small prickly shrub with dark green leaves and soft fragrant blooms. The varieties of rose used for making oil
have pink flowers.

Attributes and characteristics

Aphrodisiac, positive, tonic to
the heart, uplifting.

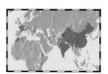

Distribution

Worldwide, but cultivated
for oil mainly in France,
Morocco, Bulgaria, China,
India.

PROPERTIES

Family name **ROSACEAE**

Method of extraction
*Steam distillation of fresh
petals, several methods of
solvent extraction, and
enfleurage.*

Chemical constituents
*Geranic (acid);
citronnellol, farnesol,
geraniol, nerol (alcohols);
eugenol (phenol); myrcene
(terpene).*

Note
Middle to base.

Aroma
*Exquisite, deep, rich, and
flowery.*

Properties
*Antidepressant,
antiphylogistic, antiseptic,
antispasmodic, antiviral,
aphrodisiac, astringent,
bactericidal, cholagogue,
choleretic, cicatrisant,
depurative, diuretic,
emmenagogue, hemostatic,
hepatic, laxative, sedative,
splenetic, stomachic, tonic.*

Blends
*Bergamot, clary sage,
geranium, jasmine,
lavender,
mandarin/tangerine,
neroli, patchouli, Roman
chamomile, sandalwood,
ylang-ylang.*

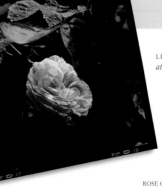

LEFT *The rose shrub bears
attractive fragrant blooms.*

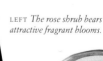

ROSE OIL

HEALTH NOTES

EFFECT ON THE SKIN

• Good for all skin conditions, especially mature, hard, dry, or sensitive skins.

PSYCHOLOGICAL AND EMOTIONAL USES

• Can help sufferers bear grief, jealousy, resentment, anger, and depression.
• A mild sedative and antidepressant, and so can be helpful at times of shock, bereavement, and melancholy.
• Eases nervous tension and stress, and lifts the heart.
• A very feminine oil, and is ideal in relationship or identity problems.

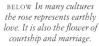

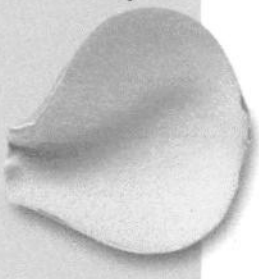

USES THROUGH THE AGES

� The Romans scattered rose petals at banquets and wore garlands of roses to prevent drunkenness. They also used them at weddings and funerals.

� It is variously believed that the rose sprung from the blood of Adonis, Venus, or Muhammad.

� Persian warriors adorned their shields with red roses.

� The rose has long been an aid to meditation and contemplation.

� The Sufi tradition holds the rose as a symbol of transcendent desire.

� The rose is a Christian representation of divine love and the symbol of the Rosacrucian order.

BELOW *In many cultures the rose represents earthly love. It is also the flower of courtship and marriage.*

� St. Dominic (1170–1221) is said to have been visited by the Virgin Mary in a mystical experience and to have received the first rosary, which had rose-scented beads.

� In the Middle Ages, Rosa gallica, the apothecaries' rose, was used as an ingredient in healing balms to treat lung disease and asthma.

🌲 Rose-flavored food was very popular in Elizabethan times.

CAUTION

Avoid during the first four months of pregnancy.

ABOVE *Legend has it that Cleopatra wore rose oil at her first meeting with Mark Antony to capture his love.*

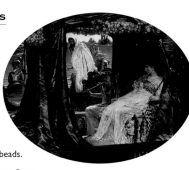

HOME USE

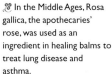

• As a tonic for the womb it can alleviate premenstrual syndrome and regulate the menstrual cycle.
• Soothes the anxiety that can cause frigidity and impotence.
• Tones the capillaries, stimulates the circulation and helps to clear any congestion.
• Balances and strengthens the digestive system.
• Can help to relieve nausea, vomiting, and constipation.
• Has a purging action on toxins and waste products.
• Can soothe sore throats and ease coughs.

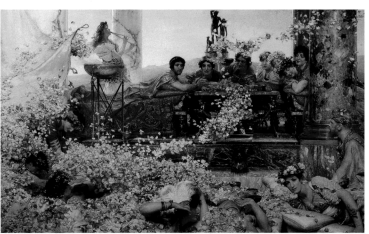

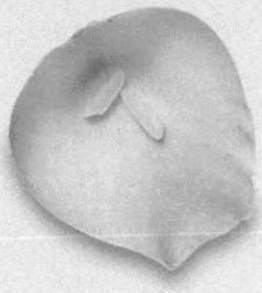

Rosemary

ROSMARINUS OFFICINALIS

In the ancient world rosemary was regarded as a sacred plant that could impart peace to both the living and the dead. In Asia it was grown on tombs so that the ancestors' help and guidance could communicate itself to the living. During the plague it was carried in neck pouches for protection against disease.

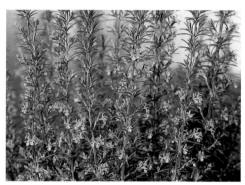

ABOVE *Rosemary's pleasant aroma makes it a welcome plant in the herb garden.*

General description

A herb with silver-green needle-shaped leaves and pale blue or lilac flowers. It is most at home near the sea (its Latin species name Rosmarinus means "dew of the sea"). The whole plant is aromatic.

Attributes and characteristics

Analgesic, protective, purifying, refreshing, stimulant.

RIGHT *Rosemary is hardy perennial herb that reaches a height of 3-6ft. (1-2m.).*

PROPERTIES

Family name LAMIACEAE (LABIATAE)

Method of extraction
Steam distilled from flowering tops and leaves.

Chemical constituents
Borneol (alcohol); cuminic (aldehyde); bornyl acetate (ester); camphor, cineole (ketones); caryophyllene (sesquiterpene); camphene, pinene (terpenes).

Note
Middle.

Aroma
Strong, clean, refreshing, and minty/herbal.

Properties
Analgesic, antidepressant, antimicrobial, antioxidant, antirheumatic, antiseptic, antispasmodic, aphrodisiac, astringent, carminative, cephalic, cholagogue, choleretic, cicatrisant, cordial, cytophylactic, digestive, diuretic, emmenagogue, fungicidal, hepatic, hypertensive, nervine, parasiticidal, resolvent, restorative, rubefacient, stimulant, stomachic, sudorific, tonic, vulnerary.

Blends
Atlas cedarwood, frankincense, geranium, ginger, grapefruit, lemongrass, lime, mandarin/tangerine, melissa/lemon balm, myrtle, sweet basil.

Distribution
Now cultivated worldwide but the most oil is produced in Morocco, France, and Spain.

USES THROUGH THE AGES

🌿 The Egyptians used it as a ritual cleansing incense. Evidence of it has been found in First Dynasty tombs.

🌿 The Greeks twisted sprigs of rosemary into their hair while studying for examinations.

🌿 Legend has it that the flowers were originally white, only turning blue when the Virgin Mary put her cloak over a bush during the Flight into Egypt.

🌿 Donna Isabella, Queen of Hungary, used it in a rejuvenating face wash that also included lemon, rose, neroli, melissa, and peppermint. "Queen of Hungary water" was made commercially in the 14th century.

🌿 It was burned in French hospitals during epidemics for its antiseptic qualities and also as an incense in French churches.

🌿 In Britain it was worn around the neck to prevent colds and wrapped around the right arm to lift the spirits. The dried leaves were put under the pillow to protect the sleeper (especially a child) against nightmares.

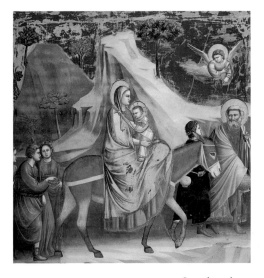

ABOVE *Legend says that the rosemary plant sheltered the Virgin Mary on her flight to Egypt.*

CAUTION

Avoid during pregnancy, if you are prone to epilepsy, or if you have high blood pressure. Do not rub or massage directly over or below varicose veins.

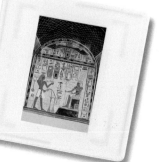

BELOW *The use of rosemary during cleansing rituals is documented in the tombs of Ancient Egypt.*

HEALTH NOTES

EFFECT ON THE SKIN
• Helps to tighten sagging skin through its astringent action.
• Good for acne, dandruff, greasy hair and skin, hair growth, and varicose veins.

PSYCHOLOGICAL AND EMOTIONAL USES
• Energizes and stimulates the central nervous system.
• Clears the head.
• Good for lethargy.
• Aids memory.
• Invigorating and stimulating.

HOME USE

• Clears headaches and migraines, especially when they are connected with gastric upset.
• A pain reliever for tired, aching muscles, especially when used in combination with sweet marjoram.
• A heart tonic and stimulant, and normalizes low blood pressure.
• Good for respiratory and chest infections.

• A liver decongestant, and can alleviate hepatitis and cirrhosis.
• Can relieve jaundice and gallstone problems.
• Eases chilblains, gout, and rheumatism, and helps with digestive problems.
• Can have a positive effect on anemia.
• Can be helpful with cellulite and edema.
• Helps alleviate water retention, scanty periods, and cramps.

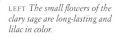

CLARY SAGE OIL

Clary sage

SALVIA SCLAREA

Although it has similar properties to common sage, clary sage is more commonly used in aromatherapy due to its lower toxicity level. It is used for treating menstrual complaints and can be very beneficial during the menopause. May also be helpful in treating throat and respiratory infections.

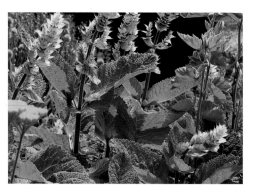

ABOVE *Clary sage is a biennial or perennial herb with large wrinkled leaves and pale violet flowers.*

PROPERTIES

Family name LABITEAE

Method of extraction
Steam distillation from green parts and flowering tops.

Chemical constituents
Linalool, salviol (alcohols); linalyl acetate (ester); cineole (ketone); caryophyllene (sesquiterpene).

Note
Top to middle.

Aroma
Nutty, strong, and heavy.

Properties
Anticonvulsive, antidepressant, antiphylogistic, antiseptic, antispasmodic, antisudorific, aphrodisiac, astringent, bactericidal, balsamic, carminative, cicatrisant, deodorant, digestive, emmenagogue, hypotensive, nervine, parturient, sedative, stomachic, tonic, uterine.

Blends
Atlas cedarwood, bergamot, cypress, frankincense, geranium, grapefruit, jasmine, juniper, lavender, lime, sandalwood.

General description

Herb with white or pale lilac flower petals that end in a hard point (skeria in Greek means "hardness"), and large, wrinkled leaves on a pink-tinged stem. The plant grows to a height of about 2ft. (60cm.).

Attributes and characteristics

Aphrodisiac, balancing, euphoric, sedative, tonic.

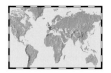

Distribution
Cultivated worldwide, the highest quality oil comes from France, Britain, and Morocco.

LEFT *The small flowers of the clary sage are long-lasting and lilac in color.*

USES THROUGH THE AGES

In 16th century England clary sage was used instead of hops in the brewing of beer. It was also used in the manufacture of German wines to make them more intoxicating.

Use of sage as a medicinal plant is recorded in ancient Egypt as a cure for infertility, and both the Greeks and the Romans thought it ensured long life.

In the Middle Ages it was known as oculus christi, meaning "the eye of Christ."

Clarus is Latin for "clear," and the herb itself (not the oil) may once have been used for clearing mucus from the eyes.

Salvia comes from the Latin salvaro or salveo, meaning "to save," that reflects the plant's "cure-all" reputation.

Clary sage oil has similar properties to common sage oil but is much safer as it contains less thujone. Take care to buy the right oil.

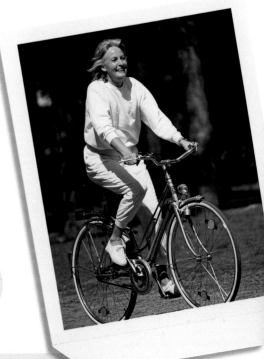

HEALTH NOTES

EFFECT ON THE SKIN
• May have regenerative properties and encourage hair regrowth.
• May also limit the production of sebum, and alleviate greasy hair and dandruff.

PSYCHOLOGICAL AND EMOTIONAL USES
• Can bring on vivid dreams and encourage clarity of dream recollection.
• Can cause a sense of euphoria, but in larger doses it can also be a narcotic and so cause drowsiness.
• Helpful in overcoming anxiety in any stressful situation.

CAUTION
Do not use it during pregnancy, although it can be beneficial once labor is very well advanced.

HOME USE

• Has an affinity with the reproductive system and is a natural balancer of the endocrine system.
• Can be very beneficial for both premenstrual syndrome and period pain, and it can help with any muscle spasms, backache, stiffness, and cramps.
• Can be greatly beneficial for any problems experienced during the menopause.

• As a uterine tonic, as well as a pain reliever, it can be beneficial in the advanced stages of labor, but should not be used any earlier.
• Can be useful for throat and respiratory infections, and it can cool skin inflammation and reduce puffiness.
• Can soothe digestive problems and ease wind, and can help with headaches, including migraines.

ABOVE *Clary sage oil may be used to treat problems experienced during the menopause.*

CAUTION
It is very sedative and likely to make concentration difficult. Large doses can cause headaches. Do not use before driving. If combined with alcohol it can cause nausea.

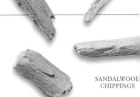

Sandalwood

SANTALUM ALBUM

SANDALWOOD
CHIPPINGS

Native to tropical Asia, sandalwood is used as a traditional incense, cosmetic, perfume, and embalming material all over the East. It has traditionally been used for building temples. Sandalwood trees are now almost extinct and are farmed in plantations exclusively for the production of oil.

SANDALWOOD OIL

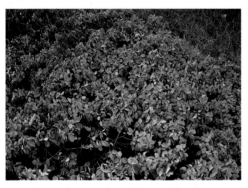

ABOVE *Oil cannot be extracted from the sandalwood tree until it is about 30 years old.*

PROPERTIES

Family name **SANTALACEAE**

Method of extraction
Distilled from dried and powered roots and heartwood.

Chemical constituents
Santalol (alcohol); furfurol (aldehyde); santalene (sesquiterpene).

Note
Base.

Aroma
Deep, woody, fruity, and exotic.

Properties
Antidepressant, antiphylogistic, antiseptic (urinary and pulmonary), antispasmodic, aphrodisiac, astringent, bactericidal, bechic, carminative, cicatrisant, diuretic, emollient, expectorant, fungicidal, insecticidal, sedative, tonic.

Blends
Bergamot, cypress, frankincense, geranium, jasmine, lavender, lemon, myrrh, neroli, rose, sweet basil, vetiver, ylang-ylang.

General description

A small evergreen tree that burrows its roots into other trees. It has a brown trunk, smooth slender branches, and pinkish flowers.

Attributes and characteristics

Aphrodisiac, elevating, purifying, relaxing.

BELOW *Sandalwood has a sensual, oriental scent, and is used extensively as a fragrance for toiletries.*

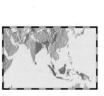

Distribution
East India (Mysore),
Taiwan, Malaysia,
Sri Lanka, Indonesia.

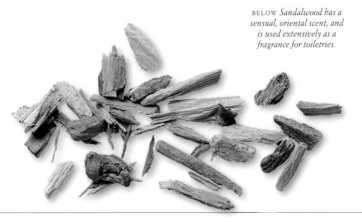

114

CAUTION

The aroma of sandalwood can linger in your clothes, even after washing.

HOME USE

• Has an affinity with the urinary tract.
• Can be massaged (in a carrier oil) into the kidney area to relieve inflammation and cystitis.
• Good for sore throats and chest infections, especially those caused by staphylococci and streptococci bacteria.
• Stimulates the immune system.

BELOW *Dab neat oil onto swollen lymph glands to fight infection and alleviate sore throats.*

• One drop can be dabbed neat onto the lymph glands under the chin if they swell during infection, and also to help a sore throat.
• May have an affinity with the reproductive system.
• Produces an ingredient that is similar to androsterone, a male hormone secreted in the armpits as a sexual signal.
• Good for heartburn and diarrhea.

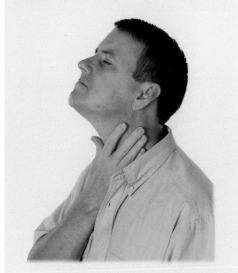

Many old temples in India are built from sandalwood, possibly because it repels white ants.

It is mentioned in the oldest texts of the Indian Veda, dating from the 5th century B.C.

It has at least 4,000 years of uninterrupted use as an aid to meditation.

It is used in a Hindu purification ceremony on the last day of the year to wash away sins. It is also combined with rose to make the famous scent aytar.

It was used by the Egyptians in the embalming process.

In Chinese medicine it is used to treat stomach ache, vomiting, gonorrhea, and skin complaints.

In Ayurveda it is a remedy for urinary and respiratory infections, and for diarrhea.

LEFT *Sandalwood is burned as an offering incense in Buddhist temples.*

Tantric philosophy recommends it to awaken the kundalini, or dormant energy at the base of the spine.

The Japanese burn it in Shinto ceremonies and at Buddhist shrines.

It is used in Tibetan medicine for insomnia and anxiety.

In Muslim countries it is burned at the feet of the recently deceased to speed their soul to heaven.

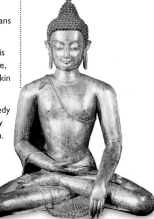

HEALTH NOTES

EFFECT ON THE SKIN
• Has a balancing and anti-inflammatory effect on dry eczema, boils, and acne.
• Can soften dry and aging skin.
• Relieves itching, especially shaving rash, and can help with dandruff.

PSYCHOLOGICAL AND EMOTIONAL USES
• An aphrodisiac and can relieve the anxiety that can lead to impotence or frigidity.
• Soothes nervous tension and anxiety.
• Can help to cut ties with the past and break obsessions.

Vetiver

VETIVERIA ZIZANOIDES

*The common name for the grass comes from the Tamil word vetiverr, meaning
"hatcheted up," referring to the method of harvesting. It is grown in India to
prevent soil erosion during the rainy season. In the East the grass is used to
keep vermin away from domestic animals.*

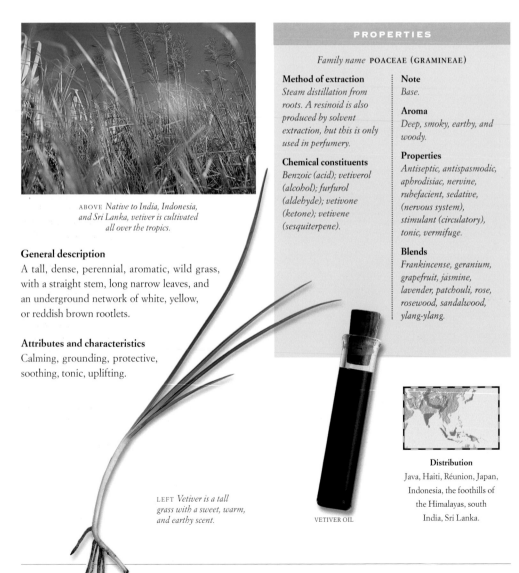

ABOVE *Native to India, Indonesia,
and Sri Lanka, vetiver is cultivated
all over the tropics.*

General description
A tall, dense, perennial, aromatic, wild grass,
with a straight stem, long narrow leaves, and
an underground network of white, yellow,
or reddish brown rootlets.

Attributes and characteristics
Calming, grounding, protective,
soothing, tonic, uplifting.

LEFT *Vetiver is a tall
grass with a sweet, warm,
and earthy scent.*

VETIVER OIL

PROPERTIES

Family name POACEAE (GRAMINEAE)

Method of extraction
*Steam distillation from
roots. A resinoid is also
produced by solvent
extraction, but this is only
used in perfumery.*

Chemical constituents
*Benzoic (acid); vetiverol
(alcohol); furfurol
(aldehyde); vetivone
(ketone); vetivene
(sesquiterpene).*

Note
Base.

Aroma
*Deep, smoky, earthy, and
woody.*

Properties
*Antiseptic, antispasmodic,
aphrodisiac, nervine,
rubefacient, sedative,
(nervous system),
stimulant (circulatory),
tonic, vermifuge.*

Blends
*Frankincense, geranium,
grapefruit, jasmine,
lavender, patchouli, rose,
rosewood, sandalwood,
ylang-ylang.*

Distribution
Java, Haiti, Réunion, Japan,
Indonesia, the foothills of
the Himalayas, south
India, Sri Lanka.

HOME USE

• Strengthens the red blood cells and promotes the transport of oxygen in the body.
• Can alleviate rheumatism, arthritis, muscular aches and pains, sprains, and stiffness, and is a tonic to the reproductive system.
• An insect repellent.

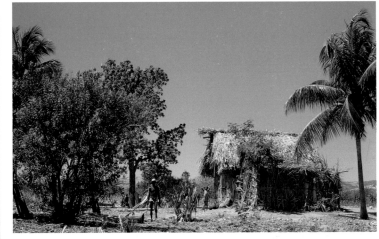

BELOW LEFT *Vetiver oil has proved to be an excellent insect repellent.*

ABOVE *The rural people of Haiti use the grass to thatch their roofs.*

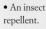

HEALTH NOTES

EFFECT ON THE SKIN
• May help with acne, cuts, oily skin, and wounds.

PSYCHOLOGICAL AND EMOTIONAL USES
• Deeply relaxing and useful for those who need to ground and center their energies.

• Has a balancing effect on the central nervous system and may be helpful for those who need to reduce their dependency on tranquilizers.
• May help deep psychological conditions.
• Helpful for mental and physical exhaustion, and for insomnia, depression, and anxiety.

USES THROUGH THE AGES

It is known as the "oil of tranquillity" in India and Sri Lanka. In Calcutta the grass is used to make awnings and sunshades that give off an aroma in the heat if sprinkled with water. Fans are also made out of it.

Sanskrit texts refer to it having been used to anoint brides.

In Ayurveda the root and essential oil are used for heatstroke, fevers, and headache.

In Russia, sachets impregnated with vetiver oil were attached to the linings of fur coats.

In Java the grass has been used for weaving mats and thatching huts, and in Haiti it has been used by the native people for thatching roofs.

A famous European perfume called Mousseline des Indes contained vetiver, sandalwood, and rose.

Sachets of powdered vetiver root, and aromatic bundles and woven screens of the grass, known as *khus khus*, are used to protect muslin from moths and insects.

Before World War II Java exported vetiver root to Europe; today it is distilled locally and is known as *akar wangi*, or "fragrant root."

In India it is grown to prevent the erosion of soil that occurs during the rainy season.

TIP

It is nontoxic, nonirritant, and nonsensitizing.

DRIED GINGER

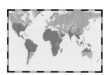

Ginger

ZINGIBER OFFICINALE

Ginger has been used as a medicinal remedy and aphrodisiac for thousands of years especially in the East. Chinese medicine uses ginger to treat many complaints and it can be found as an ingredient in many different preparations. The Ancient Greeks and Romans also included it in their medicines.

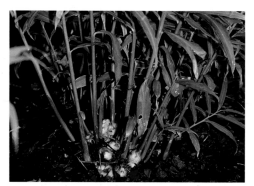

ABOVE *Grown commercially in the tropics, ginger roots are harvested in the autumn.*

PROPERTIES

Family name **ZINGIBERACEAE**

Method of extraction
Steam distilled from the rhizomes of the plant. An absolute and resinoid are also produced for the perfume industry.

Chemical constituents
Borneol (alcohol); citral (aldehyde); cineole (ketone); zingiberene (sesquiterpene); camphene, limonene, phellandrene (terpenes).

Note
Top.

Aroma
Peppery, spicy, and warm, but also fresh and pleasant.

Properties
Analgesic, antiemetic, antioxidant, antiscorbutic, antiseptic, antispasmodic, antitussive, aperitif, aphrodisiac, carminative, cephalic, expectorant, febrifuge, laxative, rubefacient, stimulant, stomachic, sudorific, tonic.

Blends
Atlas cedarwood, blue gum eucalyptus, frankincense, geranium, lemon, lime, mandarin/tangerine, neroli, patchouli, Roman chamomile, rose, rosemary, sandalwood, vetiver.

General description

It is a perennial herb with a white or yellow flowering stem and narrow dark green leaves, rising from a thick, aromatic rhizome.

Attributes and characteristics

Aphrodisiac, appetite stimulant, moisture balancer. Its action can be both warming and cooling.

Distribution
India, Malaysia, Africa, U.S.A., West Indies, and all over the tropics.

RIGHT *Ginger is a perennial herb with a thick, tuberous root.*

USES THROUGH THE AGES

❧ Throughout the ages dried ginger root has been a popular condiment, used for its taste, its smell, and its potential as a remedy against malaria.

❧ Traditional Chinese medicine uses fresh ginger to break up phlegm, to strengthen the heart, and for rheumatism, toothache, and anything to do with an imbalance of moisture.

❧ It first came to Europe via the Spice Route in the Middle Ages, and was valued during the Plague for its anti-infectious properties.

❧ The Greeks called it ziggiber, and employed it for its capability to warm the stomach and counteract the effects of poison.

❧ It is claimed that the name comes from the Gingi district in India, where ginger tea is drunk for stomach problems.

HEALTH NOTES

EFFECT ON THE SKIN
• Can help to reduce chilblains, balance the cholesterol in the blood, and, to a certain extent, alleviate varicose veins.
• Good for bruises, sores, and carbuncles.

PSYCHOLOGICAL AND EMOTIONAL USES
• Comforting, warming, and uplifting to the emotions.
• Can sharpen the senses and aid the memory.
• Both stimulating and grounding.
• A powerful nerve tonic and so is good for overtiredness, especially when used in combination with other oils.

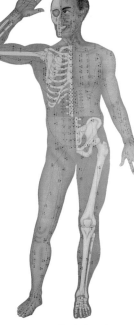

ABOVE *Fresh ginger is frequently used in Traditional Chinese Medicine.*

RIGHT *Ginger is used to alleviate morning sickness during pregnancy.*

HOME USE

• Dries out excess moisture in catarrh and runny noses, and also eases sore throats and sinusitis.
• Counteracts ailments caused by dampness, yet it can also reduce feverish conditions by encouraging the body to sweat more.
• Helpful for edema and rheumatism where warmth is required.
• Tones and settles the digestive system and stimulates the appetite, and is good to inhale both for morning sickness and travelsickness.
• Stimulates the circulation and may ease angina.

ABOVE *It helps a wide range of muscular ailments if used in massage.*

• In massage or compresses it is good for arthritic, muscular pain, including muscle cramps and spasms, and also strain and sprains, especially in the back.

CAUTION

If you have sensitive skin, be careful to dilute this oil thoroughly before use in a massage or bath.

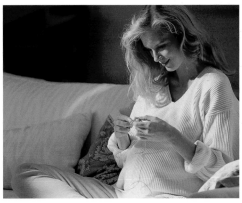

Aromatherapy in the Home

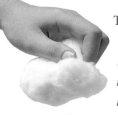

THIS SECTION *describes a variety of conditions and lists the oils that are recommended for them. The better your knowledge of the individual oils and their character, the better you will be able to choose the best oil from the lists included here. Essential oils do not work like allopathic drugs in that more than the outward symptoms need to be taken into consideration to identify the right oil or combination of oils. The character and emotional state of the person are equally relevant. You are literally marrying the character and condition of a person with the character and healing properties of a plant.*

ABOVE *Use pure cotton wool to dab a cream containing a small quantity of essential oil onto dry, greasy or combination skin*

The conditions described here, that aromatherapy can help, are grouped in the following categories: skin, hair and scalp, circulatory system, respiratory system, muscles and joints, genito-urinary system, first aid, and lastly, stress and lifestyle.

Experiment to find which of the oils recommended for each condition works best for you or the person you are treating. Always be aware of the contraindications and cautions recommended for the use of each oil. If you are treating someone for a chronic or ongoing condition or situation and you think you have the right combination of oils to help them – stick to it in your treatments for a while and then maybe try one different oil in the blend. The body builds up a tolerance for an essential oil as it might to any other substance and a variety of appropriate oils over a period of time may be just the thing. Remember that three oils are enough for a massage, bath, or compress at one time. While aromatherapy can be a very beneficial and benign way of dealing with common ailments in the home, do not hesitate to make an appointment to see your physician if you are worried about any condition.

LEFT *Aromatherapy can benefit all the family as essential oils can be used to treat a variety of complaints.*

INFORM YOUR PHYSICIAN

If you are already being treated regularly by a physician, it is best to let him or her know that you are thinking of using aromatherapy. Many physicians now recommend aromatherapy and massage, particularly in the case of stress-related conditions.

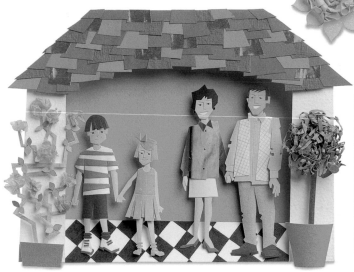

Hair and Scalp

AROMATHERAPY CAN BE *very beneficial for imbalances that occur in the hair and scalp. The scalp is obviously part of the skin itself but it can often exhibit symptoms and conditions that the rest of the skin does not manifest. Hair condition can be balanced by the use of diluted essential oils in a carrier or unscented shampoo.*

DRY OR GREASY HAIR

Greasy hair is caused by overactive sebaceous glands in the scalp, whereas dry hair occurs when the glands are underactive. Aromatherapy can regulate hair-oil production.

Make up a massage oil with a carrier oil and one or two drops of essential oil. Massage the oil into the scalp and then rinse it off. In the case of dry hair, leave the oil on the hair for a few hours or overnight before rinsing.

Oils to use
• GREASY HAIR: *Clary sage, geranium, lemon, lavender, tea tree (oil regulators); cypress, rosemary (cleansing, tonic).*
• DRY HAIR: *Roman chamomile (blonde hair); lavender, rosemary (red, brown, or black hair).*

ALOPECIA

Temporary or sudden hair loss can occur after a shock, in cases of great stress, following the birth of a child, as a symptom of an illness, or as a possible reaction to powerful medicinal drugs. Long-term hair loss and baldness are usually genetic. Aromatherapy can stimulate the scalp and help with thinning hair, but it cannot cure baldness.

The essential oils can be used in a carrier for a scalp massage: add one or two drops of essential oil to a small quantity of carrier oil, apply to the scalp, leave for half an hour, and then rinse off. Alternatively, use them in the bath or in a vaporizer.

Oils to use
• *Melissa/lemon balm, rosemary and ylang-ylang (stimulate local circulation); Atlas cedarwood and lavender (good overall tonic); clary sage, grapefruit, yarrow (promote hair growth).*

DANDRUFF

Dandruff is small dry particles of dead skin which flake off the scalp and can often be visible in the hair. It occurs when there is an imbalance of oils on the surface of the scalp, and is caused by overactive sebaceous glands, and is itchy and prone to infection.

Add one or two drops to a carrier oil, massage into the scalp, leave for half an hour, and then rinse off.

Oils to use
• *Patchouli, tea tree (anti-inflammatory, regulating, antiseptic); Atlas cedarwood, juniper, lemon, rosemary (antiseptic, astringent); geranium, lavender, sandalwood (soothing).*

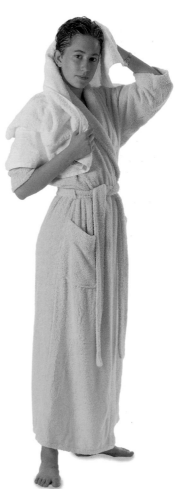

ABOVE *Add a few drops of essential oil to a carrier oil and massage into the scalp.*

Skin

MANY KINDS *of skin problems, from dry skin to dermatitis, can be helped by aromatherapy which has an integral relationship with the skin. The skin is the largest organ in the body and one of the main entry points for the oils into the body's internal systems. If the body is unhappy with an essential oil, in its quantity or usage, it will be revealed first in the skin.*

ACNE AND OILY SKIN

Acne and other forms of congested and oily skin are caused by an over-production of oil by the sebaceous glands of the skin. Bad diet, lack of exercise, hormonal imbalance, and stress can all make the problem worse. The condition also tends to be at its worst during adolescence, before or during menstruation and the menopause.

You can apply one drop of geranium, lavender, Roman chamomile, or tea tree directly to a problem area, or the oils can be used in compresses or in the bath for direct action on the skin. For stress relief, they can be vaporized in a burner or inhaled from a handkerchief.

Oils to use

• *Atlas cedarwood, bergamot, geranium, juniper, lavender, lemon, lemongrass, lime, mandarin/tangerine, myrtle, neroli, niaouli, rosemary, rosewood, sandalwood, tea tree, vetiver (antiseptic, healing, regulating); Roman chamomile (anti-inflammatory); grapefruit, lemongrass, patchouli, sweet basil (cleansing).*

DRY OR COMBINATION SKIN

Dry skin can be caused by underactive sebaceous glands or by exposure to too much sun or wind. It is prone to flaking and wrinkles more easily than greasy skin. Incessant central heating and too much alcohol can also have a drying effect and exacerbate the problem. Combination skin is a mixture of greasy and dry skin.

Use the oils in lotions and creams, in the bath, or steam your face in a basin of hot water with a towel over your head. They can also be used in a vaporizer.

Oils to use

• DRY SKIN: *Atlas cedarwood, geranium, neroli, rose, sandalwood (moisturizing); jasmine, lavender, Roman chamomile, rosewood, yarrow (sensitive skin); myrrh, patchouli, tea tree (cracked or rough skin).*

• COMBINATION SKIN: *geranium, ylang-ylang (balancing).*

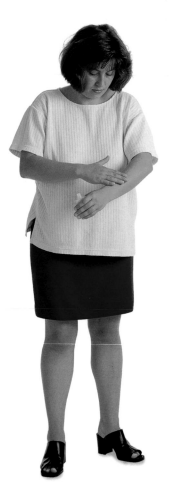

RIGHT *Blend oils with an unperfumed cream for use as a body moisturizer.*

MATURE SKIN AND WRINKLES

Young skin takes about a month to renew itself, but as the skin ages this process slows down. Stress, smoking, alcohol, pollution, sunbathing, and lack of exercise all contribute to premature aging, lack of skin moisture, and wrinkles.

Use the oils in lotions and creams, in the bath, and steam your face in a basin of hot water with a towel over your head. The oils can also be used in a vaporizer.

Oils to use

• *Clary sage, cypress, frankincense, geranium, jasmine, lavender, myrrh, neroli, patchouli, Roman chamomile, rose, rosewood, sandalwood, sweet fennel, ylang-ylang.*

SUNBURN

Sunburn should be treated as seriously as any other burn, especially as it tends to cover a wide area of the body. Lack of protection in hot sun can lead to premature aging of the skin, and to the formation of melanomas and even skin cancer. If you have any cause for concern, consult your physician. Jojoba oil has a SPF (sun protection factor) of 4, and may be used to make a light suntan lotion for day wear. You must, however, resort to commercial lotions with higher levels of protection if you plan to sunbathe. Remember to avoid angelica and bergamot oils (and possibly other citrus oils) as they can increase the photosensitivity of the skin.

Use the oils listed in cool baths, in cold compresses, or in lotions to ease sunburn.

LEFT If you do become sunburned, try a few drops of Atlas cedarwood oil in the bath, on a cold compress, or in a lotion.

Oils to use

• *Atlas cedarwood, blue gum eucalyptus, cypress, geranium, jasmine, lavender, neroli, niaouli, patchouli, Roman chamomile, rose, rosewood, sandalwood, tea tree.*

ATHLETE'S FOOT

Athlete's foot is a fungal infection of the feet. The fungus thrives on the wet floors of sports centers and swimming-pool changing-rooms and is highly contagious. The skin between the toes becomes red and itchy and starts to peel.

Use the oils in a footbath or a compress, or add a small quantity to an unscented ointment.

Oils to use

• *Lavender (antiseptic); tea tree (antifungal); geranium, myrrh, patchouli, Scotch pine (anti-inflammatory); lemongrass (deodorizing, drying).*

DERMATITIS, ECZEMA AND PSORIASIS

Skin allergies are becoming increasingly common, perhaps as a result of our ever increasingly stressful lifestyles and our polluted air, water, and food.

Use the oils in a compress, in your bathwater, or diluted in a carrier oil and stroked onto the skin. Alternatively, add one or two drops of the recommended oils to a bowl of water and steam your face in the vapor.

Oils to use

• DERMATITIS AND PSORIASIS: *Angelica, Atlas cedarwood, bergamot, cypress (soothing, anti-inflammatory); geranium, lavender, myrtle, patchouli, Roman chamomile, Scotch pine (healing).*

• ECZEMA: *geranium, juniper, niaouli, patchouli, melissa/lemon balm, myrrh (weeping eczema); sandalwood (dry eczema).*

VERRUCAS AND WARTS

Warts are small round benign tumors on the skin that are caused by a viral infection. Verrucas are warts that occur on the soles of the feet, and can be passed from person to person via the floors of sports centers and swimming-pool changing-rooms.

ABOVE Stress exacerbates all skin conditions. Bergamot oil can be vaporized in a burner to help relieve stress.

Dab a drop of oil directly onto the wart. A cotton bud is useful for this, but try not to touch the surrounding skin either with neat oil or the end of the cotton bud after you have used it, as you may either burn the skin or spread the virus.

Oils to use

• *Lemon, tea tree.*

BELOW Neat lemon oil may be used to treat verrucas and warts.

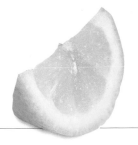

Circulatory System

THE BODY'S CIRCULATION *includes both the circulation of blood and the circulation of lymph. The blood carries oxygen and other nutrients (the products of digestion) around the body and feeds the body's organs. The lymph is the means of transport of the immune system and carries toxins and waste products out of the body. Optimum circulation can be encouraged by the use of essential oils but can also be helped by regular exercise and massage.*

CELLULITE AND WATER RETENTION

Cellulite is a build-up of toxins in the body's tissues and the glands of the lymphatic system, and can be caused both by poor circulation and fluctuating hormones. It creates a lumpy, "orange peel" texture on the thighs, buttocks, and upper arms. Cellulite and edema (water retention) frequently occur simultaneously, indicating that drainage of the body's fluid (blood and lymph) is inadequate.

Add a few drops of any of the oils listed to your bath or use them in massage toward the heart.

LEFT *Poor circulation may be improved by elevating your legs against a wall for a short period of time.*

Oils to use

• *Angelica, geranium, juniper (detoxifying); grapefruit, rosemary, mandarin/tangerine, sweet fennel (diuretic); Atlas cedarwood, cypress, lemon, lime, sandalwood, Scotch pine (circulation stimulant); lavender, patchouli (decongestant).*

SWOLLEN VEINS

This includes varicose veins, hemorrhoids, and chilblains. Abnormal swelling of veins tends to be caused by poor circulation and a loss of elasticity in the veins and their valves. This condition is initiated by a lack of exercise, standing for long periods, poor nutrition, obesity, and a sedentary lifestyle. Aromatherapy can improve the general tone of the veins, especially if combined with improved diet and gentle exercise.

Hemorrhoids are varicose veins that are located just above the opening of the anus. They are often caused by a restriction of the normal circulation of blood to the rectum. This can occur temporarily during pregnancy, or may be a permanent symptom of liver disease or chronic constipation. Pain and discomfort from hemorrhoids can encourage constipation, so the two conditions aggravate each another.

Chilblains are swollen, discolored veins on the fingers, toes, and backs of the legs that may appear after exposure to very cold weather.

Use the oils in the bath, in compresses, in a mild local wash, or in a vaporizer. Treat the affected areas very gently and do not apply any pressure to them.

Oils to use

• VARICOSE VEINS: *Cypress, ginger, juniper, lavender, lemon, lime, myrrh, rosemary, Scotch pine, sweet basil, sweet marjoram, tea tree, yarrow.*
• HEMORRHOIDS: *Bergamot, clary sage, cypress, frankincense, geranium, juniper, lemon, myrrh, myrtle, neroli, niaouli, patchouli, Roman chamomile, sandalwood, tea tree. Use rosemary, sweet fennel and sweet marjoram if you are also constipated.*
• CHILBLAINS: *Blue gum eucalyptus, ginger, sweet basil; cypress, juniper, lemon, lemongrass, rosemary, sweet marjoram, tea tree, yarrow.*

Muscles and Joints

MUSCULAR AND JOINT pain can affect many parts of the body. The use of essential oils in massage, in the burner, and in the bath can literally ease muscle tension and encourage the elimination of waste products, including the build-up of toxins that can be a cause of rheumatism. Aromatherapy can also help with any physical tensions and pains that are stress-related.

CRAMP

Muscle spasm can be caused by too much exercise, poor circulation, or vitamin deficiency, or can accompany the beginning of a period. Use of essential oils can help in relaxing the tension and easing the pain. As cramp often strikes at night, they can also help you get back to sleep.

Use the oils in the burner or dab them on your pillow for relaxation, use them in a compress or massage for pain relief, or use them in the bath for both.

Oils to use
• *Blue gum eucalyptus, ginger, grapefruit, niaouli, rosemary, sweet marjoram, vetiver (warming, pain relieving); cypress, lemon, mandarin/tangerine, rose, Scotch pine, sweet basil (stimulate the circulation); clary sage, jasmine, juniper, sweet fennel (relief from period pain); lavender, Roman chamomile, ylang-ylang (relaxing).*

BACKACHE

Backache will affect many people at some time in their lives. It can be caused by overexercising, poor posture, lifting heavy weights, or using muscles that have not been warmed up properly. Even the tiniest mistake can be the catalyst for days or even weeks of back pain and discomfort.

Use the oils in the bath, in a massage for local physical effect, in the burner, or put a drop on your bedclothes for a good night's sleep.

Oils to use
• *Juniper, Roman chamomile, rosemary, sweet basil (soothing, stimulating); Blue gum eucalyptus, niaouli, Scotch pine, sweet marjoram, vetiver (relaxing, warming); lavender, clary sage (relaxing, anti-inflammatory).*

BELOW *Remember to warm up muscles properly before strenuous physical exercise.*

RHEUMATISM AND ARTHRITIS

Rheumatism is pain and inflammation in the muscles, ligaments, and connective tissues of the joints. Oils can help to alleviate suffering by easing muscles, bringing down swelling, and lessening pain.

Use the essential oils in carrier oil in a massage (all over or local), in a vaporizer, in compresses, or add them to the bathwater. They can also be inhaled from handkerchiefs or bedclothes.

Oils to use
• *Blue gum eucalyptus, ginger, lavender, juniper, Roman chamomile, Scotch pine, sweet marjoram, vetiver (warming and relaxing); angelica, cypress, lemon, lime, myrrh, rosemary, sweet basil, yarrow (anti-inflammatory).*

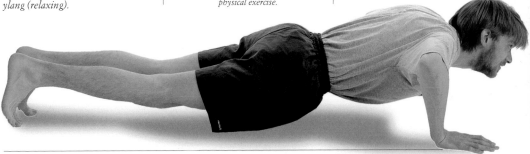

Genito-Urinary System

SOME ESSENTIAL *oils show a particular affinity with the genito-urinary system, and careful use may alleviate painful or irritating conditions. Problems that can be helped by the use of essential oils tend to be either cases of inflammation, such as cystitis, or imbalance, as in the case of candida albicans where the balance of certain yeasts in the body is disturbed.*

ABOVE *Use essential oils as an effective remedy for painful and irritating genito - urinary complaints*

CYSTITIS

Cystitis is an inflammation of the bladder and is most frequently caused by a bacterial infection. It is far more common in women than men, and is characterized by the frequent and painful passing of urine. If the right oils are used at the first sign of infection a full-blown case of cystitis can often be avoided.

Use as a local wash in mild dilution, in a compress, or in the bath.

Oils to use
• *Angelica, Atlas cedarwood, blue gum eucalyptus, frankincense, juniper, lavender, niaouli, Roman chamomile, sandalwood, tea tree.*

THRUSH

The *Candida albicans* organism is a kind of yeast that lives inside us all. It becomes a problem only if it spreads outside the gut. Excessive *Candida* may occur following a course of antibiotics as these can kill the bacteria in the gut that normally keep it under control. The commonest symptom of excessive *Candida* is thrush, an infection of the mucus membranes of the genital area or, sometimes, the mouth (particularly common in babies).

Tea tree is the best oil to use because of its powerful antifungal, antiviral, and antiseptic properties. Dilute one or two drops in a bowl of warm water and bathe the genital area. Use the other oils in the bath or vaporizer.

Oils to use
• *Juniper, lavender, tea tree (antifungal); myrrh, sandalwood (antiseptic).*

GENITAL HERPES

Genital herpes is a virus spread by sexual contact. It is caused by the Herpes Simplex II Virus, that may, in fact, be the same virus as Herpes Simplex I virus (that causes cold sores). Small painful blisters appear in the genital region and may last up to several weeks.

Use the oils in a very mild local wash with boiled (and cooled) water. Bergamot is useful because of its affinity with the genito-urinary system and because it is an excellent oil for stress relief and depression, making it an even more apt choice for this condition.

Oils to Use:
• *Bergamot, Eucalyptus, Lavender, Tea Tree.*

Respiratory System

CERTAIN ESSENTIAL oils can help to ease any muscle spasm that occurs in the body's breathing apparatus, whether caused by tension, an allergy, or by a virus. Others can work to clear any excess mucus from the body. Particles of essential oil travel in the air toward the lungs and can help to clear an airway through any obstruction in their path.

HAYFEVER

Hayfever is an allergy that affects the eyes, the throat, and the lining of the nose. It causes a runny nose, sneezing, and streaming eyes whenever the pollen that causes the allergy is in the air.

Use the oils in a vaporizer or in the bath.

Oils to use

• *Blue gum eucalyptus, ginger, lavender, myrrh, myrtle, sweet basil (for the symptoms); melissa/lemon balm, Roman chamomile (for the cause of the allergic reaction).*

ASTHMA AND BREATHING PROBLEMS

Asthma is caused by muscle spasm in the small air passages of the lungs, and is characterized by wheezing and shortness of breath. Because the air passages are narrowed, mucus builds up in the lungs, thereby making it increasingly difficult for the sufferer to breathe. Asthma can be caused by an allergic reaction, for example to dust or animal hair, it may be preceded by an infection, or it may be stress related. It may also be brought on by over-exercise.

Consult your physician if you think you may have had your first asthma attack or if you are experiencing any difficulty in breathing.

Use the oils in a vaporizer, as an inhalation, as a chest rub (one or two drops in carrier oil), in a full-body massage, in the bath, in a compress, or inhale them straight out of the bottle (in moderation).

Oils to use

• *Angelica, cypress, melissa/lemon balm, myrrh, rosewood, sweet fennel (coughing); Atlas cedarwood, bergamot, clary sage, jasmine, lavender, Roman chamomile, sandalwood, sweet marjoram (soothing, calming); blue gum eucalyptus, frankincense, lemon, lime, myrtle, niaouli, (decongestant); rosemary, Scotch pine, tea tree (antiviral); sweet basil (antiallergenic); geranium (tonic).*

COLDS AND FLU

Both colds and flu are caused by an array of different viruses. Symptoms include fever, sweating, aching, sneezing, coughing, tiredness, a sore throat, and chest congestion.

Use the oils in a vaporizer, a warm bath, on your bedclothes, or in a chest rub.

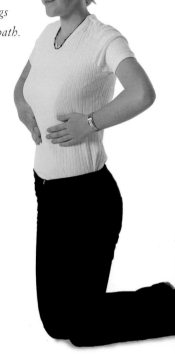

ABOVE *Breathing exercises, together with the use of essential oils, may alleviate respiratory problems.*

Oils to use

• *Angelica, Atlas cedarwood, blue gum eucalyptus, frankincense, myrrh, niaouli, Scotch pine, sweet marjoram, tea tree (decongestant, expectorant); cypress, rosemary, sweet fennel (antispasmodic); geranium, lavender, rosewood, sandalwood (antiseptic); ginger, lemon, lime, melissa/lemon balm, yarrow (febrifuge).*

First Aid

SUPERFICIAL *(but nevertheless painful) burns and also bruises and bites can often be quickly treated with essential oils to bring almost instant relief. Gattefossé, the French pharmacist plunged his burnt hand into a bowl of neat lavender oil and discovered its powerful healing properties. Lavender is not the only oil to use, but its wide range of properties make it the "rescue remedy" of the essential oils, and, if you only carry one oil with you, this is the oil to carry. Tea tree oil, too, has powerful cleansing and healing properties. Remember, if you are choosing which oil to use in a particular situation, look at the other relevant factors acting upon the situation. How is the injured person feeling?*

BITES AND STINGS

The external effects of insect bites and stings can be greatly alleviated by the application of essential oils. The antiseptic and anti-inflammatory properties of several oils can frequently bring relief from itching and inflammation. This is one of the occasions when you can use a drop of neat lavender or tea tree oil directly onto the affected area. Use the other oils in the bath or a cold compress, especially if there are several or many bites, as can be the case with mosquito bites. If you are at all worried about someone seek immediate medical care.

CAUTION

Remember to seek medical advice if the person affected has a high temperature or a fever. Some people can have severe allergic attacks to, for example, bee stings..

Oils to use

• *Geranium, lavender, melissa/ lemon balm, niaouli, sweet basil, sweet fennel, tea tree (soothing, anti-inflammatory, antiseptic).*

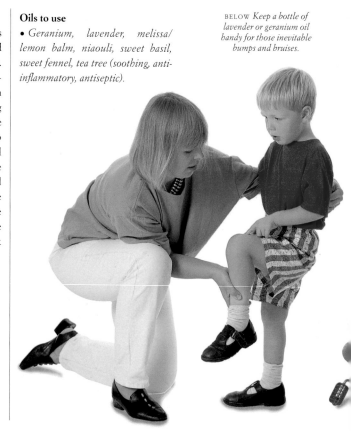

BELOW *Keep a bottle of lavender or geranium oil handy for those inevitable bumps and bruises.*

BRUISES

Bruises indicate mild tissue damage, usually caused by a bump or a knock, and can be accompanied by local swelling and pain. Blood seeping from the capillaries can cause discoloration of the skin. The skin becomes bluish-black in color, before fading to yellowish-brown. People who have an obvious and frequent tendency to bruise easily should seek medical advice as this can indicate a kidney disorder or a vitamin C deficiency.

The oils are best used in a cold compress, especially initially, and a drop of lavender oil or geranium oil can be dabbed directly on the bruise. The various oils recommended can also be used in the bath, especially for bruising over a wide area and also in massage when the bruise has faded to a greenish yellow color, to increase local circulation in order to complete the healing process.

Oils to use

• *Clary sage, ginger, rosemary, sweet fennel (warming, increase circulation); geranium, myrtle, sweet marjoram (soothing); cypress, lavender (anti-inflammatory).*

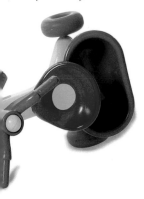

INSECT REPELLENTS

Several essential oils are excellent repellents of insects of all kinds. The oils can be used on the skin in a blend with a carrier oil or in the case of lavender oil you can apply the oil neat to the skin in moderation.

Essential oils can be made into a home made spritzer or personal body spray or into a room spray if diluted with distilled or mineral water and an alcohol such as vodka. Personal body sprays can be made using the recipe for toners. Refer to Homemade Toiletries, *see page 30.*

You can also use the oils in the bath or in a cold compress or you could even make an insect repellent, aromatic moisturizing skin cream. Refer again to Homemade Toiletries.

Another simple way to utilize the insect repellent oils is to use them in any sort of burner in any room where you want to be. You can also dab lavender oil on bed clothes or on a mosquito net if you are traveling in a hot country to discourage any irritating or harmful insects around.

Oils to use

• *Atlas Cedarwood, bergamot, blue gum eucalyptus, cypress, geranium, lavender, lemon, lemongrass, rosewood, sweet basil, vetiver.*

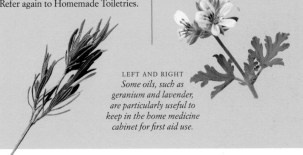

LEFT AND RIGHT
Some oils, such as geranium and lavender, are particularly useful to keep in the home medicine cabinet for first aid use.

MILD BURNS

Burns and scalds are caused by the skin coming into contact with something hot and result in a sensitive area or blister that becomes vulnerable to infection.

Immediately immerse the area in cold water or apply a cold compress to cool the area down and keep it clean. Do not apply cream, oil, or butter as this can encourage infection and retain the heat. One drop of lavender or tea tree can be dropped onto a burn as a first-aid measure immediately after the accident. You can also sprinkle one or

CAUTION
If the burn is serious, consult your nearest hospital emergency room.

two drops of either these oils or niaouli onto a gauze pad and lay it over the blister. The other oils listed can be used in a cold compress.

Oils to use

• *Blue gum eucalyptus, lavender, niaouli, tea tree (soothing, healing, antiseptic); geranium, Roman chamomile, rose (soothing, healing).*

Stress and Lifestyle

OUR MODERN, *frequently stress-filled lives leave us prone to exhaustion or insomnia, depression, and digestive problems. Essential oils can help with any of the symptoms of modern living, whether it is inadequate diet, overindulging in social or self destructive activities, stress, or exhaustion brought on by rushing around the world. The oils can act as a pick-me-up, a destressing agent, an aid to restful sleep, and an antacid – all properties that may stop you rushing into the pharmacist for a quick fix or cure.*

DEPRESSION

Everyone feels depressed or down in the dumps at some time. Whatever the causes, the oils used in aromatherapy can help. This is partly because smells register in the same part of your brain as memories, moods, and emotions.

Use the essential oils in a relaxing or stimulating bath or in the vaporizer. They can also be inhaled direct from the bottle (ylang-ylang oil works particularly well when used in this way).

Oils to use

• *Atlas cedarwood, bergamot, cypress, frankincense, geranium, grapefruit, jasmine, juniper, lavender, lemongrass, lime, mandarin/tangerine, melissa/lemon balm, myrrh, myrtle, neroli, patchouli, Roman chamomile, rose, rosemary, rosewood, sandalwood, Scotch pine, sweet marjoram, vetiver, yarrow, ylang-ylang.*

LEFT *Painful headaches or migraines may be relieved by the use of soothing oils.*

DIGESTIVE PROBLEMS

Digestive problems include indigestion, constipation, diarrhea, and irritable bowel syndrome (IBS). They can be caused by stress and an unhealthy diet: eating too much or too quickly, eating too little or too irregularly, eating too little fiber or too much rich food – or worrying too much about all of these things.

Use the oils in the bath, massage, a vaporizer, or in compresses.

Oils to use

• INDIGESTION: *Angelica, bergamot, frankincense, ginger, lavender, lemongrass, lime, mandarin/tangerine, myrrh, niaouli, Roman chamomile, rose, rosemary, sandalwood, sweet basil, sweet fennel, yarrow.* DIARRHEA: *Ginger, myrtle, Roman chamomile, sandalwood, sweet fennel, sweet marjoram, yarrow.* CONSTIPATION: *Ginger, juniper, lemongrass, lemon, mandarin/tangerine, Roman chamomile, rosemary, sweet basil, sweet fennel.* IBS: *Lavender, melissa/lemon balm, neroli, Roman chamomile, sweet fennel, sweet marjoram.*

EXHAUSTION

Sometimes when you've been working or playing too hard, oils can act as a pick-me-up to keep you going until you can get the rest and relaxation your body and mind need.

Use the oils in a bath, in a vaporizer, or in a face and neck massage.

Oils to use
• *Angelica, blue gum eucalyptus, ginger, grapefruit, juniper, lemon, lemongrass, lime, mandarin/tangerine, niaouli, rosemary, Scotch pine, tea tree (stimulating); bergamot, clary sage, jasmine, myrtle, sweet basil (uplifting, euphoric); frankincense, geranium, lavender, myrrh, patchouli, Roman chamomile, rosewood, sweet fennel, ylang-ylang (relaxing).*

HEADACHES AND MIGRAINES

A headache is a sign that your body has had enough. Resting in a dark room may alleviate it.

Use the oils in a vaporizer, in the bath, or in a scalp or facial massage.

Oils to use
• *Angelica, blue gum eucalyptus, juniper, lemongrass, rosemary (clear the head); lavender, Roman chamomile, rose, rosemary, sweet marjoram (for pain relief and relaxation); clary sage, frankincense, lemon, melissa/lemon balm (relieve tension).*

RIGHT *Pain caused by excessive alcohol intake may be relieved with oils such as geranium or lavender*

HANGOVER

Essential oils can relieve a headache and feelings of nausea, clear the head, and banish the apathy that accompanies a hangover.

Use the oils in the bath or in a massage, put them in a vaporizer, or make a cold compress for your forehead – and drink lots of water!

Oils to use
• *Geranium, lavender, neroli, rose (for the headache and apathy); angelica, ginger, lemon, lime (to clear the head and relieve the nausea).*

INSOMNIA

Inability to sleep can be caused by stress and anxiety, and quickly leads to overtiredness, nervous irritability, and an inability to cope. Essential oils can help you break the cycle.

Use the oils in the bath or vaporize them in your bedroom.

Oils to use
• *Bergamot, cypress, geranium, jasmine, lavender, mandarin/tangerine, melissa/lemon balm, myrtle, neroli, Roman chamomile, rose, sandalwood, sweet marjoram, vetiver, yarrow, ylang-ylang.*

JETLAG AND TRAVELSICKNESS

Disorientation, swollen ankles, dehydration, loss of appetite, and confusion caused by a change of time zone are all symptoms of jetlag. Travel sickness takes the form of nausea caused either by motion, or fear of the journey itself.

Inhale the oils from the bottle, a handkerchief, or vaporizer, or use them in the bath or a massage.

Oils to use
• JETLAG: *Bergamot, blue gum eucalyptus, grapefruit, lemon, lemongrass, rosemary (reviving); geranium, juniper, lavender, neroli, Roman chamomile, rosewood, vetiver (calming and reassuring); Atlas cedarwood, cypress (reduce swelling).*
• TRAVELSICKNESS: *Angelica, ginger, lemon, mandarin/ tangerine, rosewood, sweet fennel, sweet marjoram (to settle the stomach); bergamot, frankincense, sandalwood (soothing, uplifting).*

Aromatherapy for Women, Children, and the Elderly

THERE ARE MANY *reasons why the healing powers and special affinities of essential oils can have specific relevance to women, children, and the elderly. With care, the oils can be safely used from the beginning to the end of life and certain oils have special application for women during menstruation, pregnancy, and the menopause.*

AROMATHERAPY AND MENSTRUATION

If you have painful, uncomfortable, scanty, or heavy periods, aromatherapy can help on both an emotional level and physical level.

Use the essential oils in your bathwater, in a vaporizer, in massage, or in compresses.

Oils to use

• PREMENSTRUAL SYNDROME: *Frankincense, geranium, grapefruit, lavender, mandarin/tangerine, melissa/lemon balm, neroli, rose, Roman chamomile, sandalwood, vetiver (calming and/or hormone-balancing); bergamot, clary sage, jasmine, juniper (emotionally uplifting); cypress, patchouli, rosemary, sweet fennel (reduce fluid retention).*
• PAINFUL PERIODS: *Clary sage, cypress, geranium, ginger, juniper, lavender, Scotch pine, sweet basil, sweet fennel, sweet marjoram, vetiver.*
• SCANTY OR HEAVY PERIODS: *Clary sage, juniper, lavender, melissa/lemon balm, myrrh, Roman chamomile, rose, rosemary, sweet fennel, sweet marjoram, yarrow.*

BATH TIME

If you like to have your children in the bath with you, take your vaporizer into the bathroom, or use only the smallest quantities of the most gentle and safest oils for your children.

AROMATHERAPY FOR CHILDREN AND BABIES

Aromatherapy oils can safely be used in a vaporizer for the benefit of children and even babies. The best oils to introduce your child to are mandarin, myrtle, lavender, and Roman chamomile. They should all be used via a vaporizer. Do not use the oils in the bath or directly on a child's skin until he or she is at least 12 months old; even then, only use one drop in a small quantity of carrier oil.

Massaging your baby with plain oil can be a wonderful bonding experience. There are many baby massage courses around, and the International Association of Infant Massage has registered teachers in most countries.

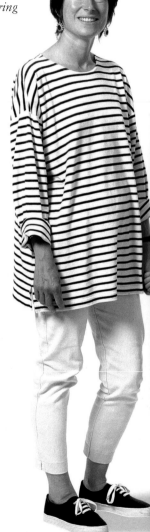

CAUTION

Before using even the gentlest oils on your child, carry out a patch test first (*see page 18*). You should always perform a test before introducing each new oil.

AROMATHERAPY AND THE MENOPAUSE

Some women sail through the menopause with little or no disturbance to their outward lives, while others experience depression, irregular and heavy periods, hot flushes, and other symptoms, sometimes spread over several years. As well as problems caused by hormonal changes, at the time of her menopause every woman has to confront a number of issues, reassessing and analyzing the choices she has made in her life so far.

The suggested oils can be used in the bath, in vaporizers, and in massage. The loving touch of a professional therapist, partner, or family member can be particularly valuable at this time.

CAUTION

It is important to avoid rosemary oil and Scotch pine oil if you have high blood pressure

LEFT *Aromatherapy oils can be particularly beneficial for women, children, and the elderly.*

Oils to use

• *Bergamot, lemon, mandarin/tangerine, neroli, sandalwood, ylangylang (emotionally uplifting); clary sage, cypress, frankincense, geranium, jasmine, Roman chamomile, sweet fennel (supportive with hormonal changes); melissa/lemon balm, rose, Scotch pine, sweet marjoram (both).*

AROMATHERAPY AND THE ELDERLY

There is absolutely no reason why you cannot enjoy aromatherapy massage right into old age. If a full-body massage does not appeal then why not try a relaxing aromatherapy foot, hand, or face massage from a professional therapist or a member of your family? Remember that a good qualified professional therapist will always be happy to talk to you about what you want. Alternatively, you can easily use essential oils in a vaporizer, in a handkerchief, or on your pillow at night. If you enjoy using essential oils in the bath, make sure that they are mixed thoroughly into the bathwater and avoid those that can irritate sensitive skin (*see* the precautions and contraindications in the Materia Medica section).

FLASHBACKS

The evocative scents of essential oils often help to bring back memories. Recounting your life experiences while you have your feet, hands, face, neck, and shoulders massaged by a friend or relative is a wonderful way to spend an afternoon.

Aromatherapy in Pregnancy and Childbirth

THROUGHOUT PREGNANCY *and during the birth itself certain oils can be thoroughly supportive. These are the oils that can become friends and help you every step of the way as your welcome your baby into the world. Use the oils for your pleasure and support and to ease any discomfort that you may be experiencing but do not hesitate to turn to other methods if that is what you feel you need. This is your time and your new baby's time.*

DURING PREGNANCY

The benefits of some essential oils can be enjoyed throughout your pregnancy. Use them in a vaporizer as you are falling asleep, while you are enjoying a relaxing bath, or during a plain oil massage. However, several essential oils are emmenagogues (likely to restore menstrual bleeding) and some might raise your blood pressure. Essential oils to avoid until you are in your fifth month and the pregnancy is well established include Atlas cedarwood, clary sage, cypress, jasmine, juniper, lavender, myrrh, rose, rosemary, sweet basil, sweet fennel, and sweet marjoram.

It is better to use the oils recommended for pregnancy only in a vaporizer and not on your skin unless you are using them under the supervision of a properly qualified professional therapist. You and your baby are so sensitive at this time that although many oils may be perfectly safe to use, especially in minute quantities, it is still best to reserve them for the burner.

Massage is also best avoided until the fifth month of the pregnancy, but after that it can make you feel good by soothing away tensions, irritations, and fatigue. Many professional massage therapists are experienced in the physical and emotional challenges that pregnancy brings, and will ensure that you are comfortably positioned during a massage. However, at this special time you may prefer the loving touch and attention of a massage by your partner. Refer to The Art of Massage (*see page 40*) for details of massage techniques during pregnancy.

CAUTION
Avoid any essential oil not mentioned in this book. If you have any doubts or queries, consult a professional therapist.

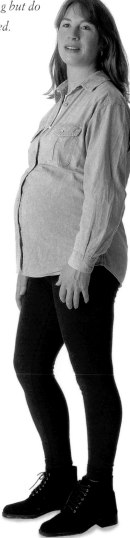

RIGHT *Take care which oils you use during pregnancy. Choose those that are non-toxic and non-irritating.*

DURING LABOR

Once you are in labor, essential oils can be very supportive. Frankincense, geranium, lavender, rose, and ylang-ylang can be lovely in a vaporizer in the early stages, and neroli can be especially beneficial if you are feeling at all apprehensive. Once you are well dilated and labor is advanced, jasmine and clary sage can be extremely useful as they are both euphoric, pain relievers, and tonics to the uterus.

However much you may want an aromatic birth, you may find that every essential oil you love makes you feel nauseous once labor actually starts. If this happens, simply don't use them. Recent research at Warwick University in the U.K. has found that if you don't like the smell of an essential oil, even temporarily, your central nervous system will block the therapeutic properties of that particular oil.

FEEL PAMPERED

Regular massage can help alleviate tension in the lower back, the neck, or wherever else you might be feeling it. It can also improve the circulation and the lymph flow, and it can give you the opportunity to relax and feel pampered and supported.

AFTER THE BIRTH

In the period following the birth you can use essential oils to give you support. Treat yourself to your favorite oils in a vaporizer: this is the time for a single drop of the expensive oils jasmine, neroli, or rose to make you feel special, while ylang-ylang can also be very beneficial. If you are having trouble with the flow of your breast milk, try sweet fennel or lemongrass oil compresses, but be sure to wipe the oil off thoroughly.

TIP

Remember that with babies in particular your smell is the only aromatherapy they need, in combination with your loving touch.

CAUTION

Don't let any essential oil get into your baby's mouth.

MISCARRIAGE

If you lose a baby during pregnancy for any reason there can be a very difficult emotional journey ahead and aromatherapy can be a great help and support to those who are grieving. The powerful and luxurious oils of neroli, rose, and jasmine, or indeed any other oil that you find particularly attractive at this time, can be used to great advantage, whether you use the oils privately at home or go to a therapist. The loving touch and understanding of a friend, a partner, or a sympathetic therapist can be incredibly beneficial. Indulge yourself and give yourself time to try to relax and benefit from the therapeutic vapors of these wonderful oils.

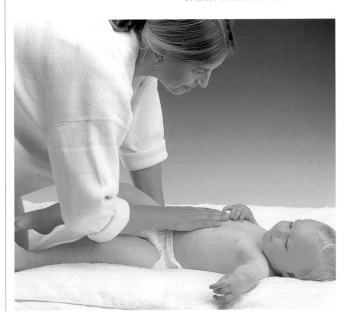

RIGHT *Babies love the touch of their mother's hands and will greatly enjoy a gentle massage.*

135

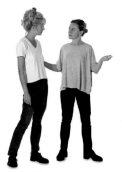

Visiting a Therapist

THE BEST WAY *to find a good professional therapist is through personal recommendation. If, however, you do not know anyone who can recommend a therapist, go to a holistic health center; they will have a great many well-trained therapists on their registers.*

ABOVE *You may visit a therapist at his or her home or in a health center.*

The first time you visit an aromatherapist he or she will ask you several questions about your health and lifestyle, and what you need from the treatment. When the therapist is satisfied that he or she has gained enough information to blend the right oils for you, you will be asked to undress and told to lie on the treatment couch. The therapist may leave the room while you do this, or he or she may stay and prepare the oils. A good holistic massage is likely to involve a complete treatment of the whole body, although any specific needs and requests you may have can be respected and incorporated.

Some therapists lift and stretch your limbs or your neck in the course of the treatment. Feel free to tell them if they are doing anything that you do not find pleasant. If they want you to do anything to help they will ask. Otherwise, just lie back and relax. The therapist may ask for feedback during the treatment on whether the pressure is firm enough or too firm. Some therapists play soothing and relaxing music, others do not.

If you have any questions on your treatment or aromatherapy in general, feel free to ask the therapist before, during, or, briefly, after the treatment. You may wish to ask what oils are being used and why they have been chosen for you. You can also request your therapist to use certain essential oils, although exposure to new ones may give you a different insight into your physical condition or state of mind.

Aromatherapy massage is often very gentle (to ensure the oils are absorbed by the skin as much as to relax tense muscles), but you can always ask for a stronger treatment. Remember, however, that a massage treatment should be thoroughly pleasurable – even if you have knotted muscles, the removal of tension should not be unpleasant. If you feel uncomfortable, don't hesitate to say so.

In some health centers you may be given the opportunity to relax for a while after the treatment in order to absorb the beneficial effects. Other therapists want you to leave fairly quickly as they may have another client waiting.

You will be required either to pay the therapist directly or to pay the receptionist at the center. Some individual therapists or centers give discounts if you book several treatments or pay for them in advance. If you wish to receive treatments from a particular therapist on a regular basis, you should ask if this can be arranged. For your first treatment it is a good idea to book a 90-minute session, although subsequently you may find you prefer more frequent 60-minute treatments.

If you would like to visit an independent therapist at his or her home or if you want them to come to your home, speak with them on the telephone first so you can see how you feel about each other. Some therapists, even if they like to work from home or are happy to come to your home, may prefer you to come to a health center for your first treatment. That way you can decide if you want to work together, without the worry of trespassing on the other's private space.

CAUTION

If you feel wobbly, vulnerable, or lightheaded it is best not to drive straight after a treatment. Drink some water or a warm beverage (avoid tea, coffee, and alcohol) and take a rest before you get in your car.

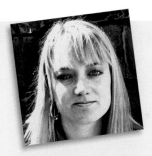

Jane Smith is a 25-year-old secretary. Although generally in good health, she has been unable to sleep properly for the last few weeks. She realizes that she is suffering from stress and hopes that aromatherapy will help her to relax.

The therapist needs a holistic understanding of your condition, and you should try to be as honest and thorough as possible when answering questions.

The health problems of your family members are often highly relevant to an understanding of your own health, and will help the therapist to choose the right treatment.

Illnesses and ailments that affect you can indicate the physical areas and body systems to which the therapist should pay particular attention.

CASE STUDY

TREATMENT RECORD

Name **Jane Smith**   Height **5'6"**
Phone number **0121 924 1111**   Weight **10 stone**
Address **62 Edgbaston St.**   Date of birth **25/9/72**
Edgbaston

Name/address/phone number of GP **Ms Jones   Surgery 0121 924 2222**
When did you last visit your GP **don't remember**   Why? **Vaccinztion**
Who were you referred by? **A friend**
What do you want from your treatment? **Relaxation**
Social/marital/family status **Single**
Occupation/pastimes (including sports, hobbies, current jobs) **Secretary – tennis, walking**

Please answer as thoroughly as possible

- How would you describe your general state of health
  Good
- How would you describe your diet?
  Varied
- Are you undergoing any other form of treatment/therapy?
  No
- Do you often get coughs, colds or sore throats?
  Yes
- Have you been abroad lately, if so where?
  No
- Do you wear glasses/contact lenses or a hearing aid?
  Yes – glasses
- Have you had an X-ray or hospital visit in the past 3 years?
  No

- Do you have an particular problems at the moment?
  No
- On a stress scale of 1(low) to 10(high) where do you fit?
  7
- Are you taking any medication at the moment?
  No
- What is your skin type (oily, dry?)
  dry
- Could you be pregnant? When was your last period?
  No   ?
- Do you smoke? How many each day?
  No
- Have you had any surgery?
  No

Do you or does anyone in your immediate family have any history or current experience of (answer yes or no):

Migranes	**No**	Heart problems	**No**	High/low blood pressure	**No**	Thrombosis	**No**
Diabetes	**No**	Chest problems	**No**	Kidney problems	**No**	Varicose veins	**No**
Epilepsy	**No**	Allergies	**Yes**	Bladder problems	**No**	Hepatitis	**No**

Give brief details **mum – strawberries**

Do you ever get (answer yes or no):

Insomnia	**Yes**	Backache	**Yes**	Ulcers	**No**	Bronchitis **No**	Chill blains **No**
Asthma	**No**	Arthritis	**No**	Cold hands and feet **Yes**	Eczema **Yes**	Constipation **No**
Cystitis	**Yes**	Other skin problems **No**	Heartburn **No**	Period pains **No**	Hay fever **No**

Give brief details **Occasional eczema, + cold hands in winter Frequent mild cystitis**

Do you have any injuries, illnesses or chronic ailments not covered elsewhere in this treatment record
No

Is there anything else I might need to know **No**

Please sign and date it
Jane Smith

Declaration: I will inform the therapist of any condition which may arise during my course of treatment which has not been covered above

ABOVE *Your therapist will ask you questions about your general health and lifestyle.*

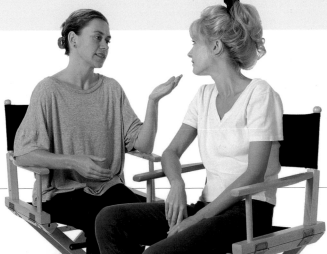

LEFT *You should feel trust in your therapist and be able to talk comfortably with him or her.*

Properties of Essential Oils

ABORTIFACIENT Can cause a miscarriage.

ANALGESIC Pain relieving.

ANAPHRODISIAC Diminishing sexual desire.

ANESTHETIC Loss of sensation; pain relieving.

ANODYNE Stills pains and quietens disturbed feelings.

ANTACID Combats acid imbalance.

ANTIALLERGENIC Reduces symptoms of allergy.

ANTIANEMIC Combats anemia.

ANTIARTHRITIC Combats arthritis.

ANTIBILIOUS Helps to remove excess bile from the body.

ANTIBIOTIC Destroys or prevents the growth of bacteria.

ANTICATARRHAL Helps remove excess catarrh from the body.

ANTICOAGULANT Prevents blood from clotting.

ANTICONVULSIVE Helps control convulsions.

ANTIDEPRESSANT Uplifting; counteracts melancholy.

ANTIDIARRHEAL Combats diarrhea.

ANTIDONTALGIC Relieves toothache.

ANTIEMETIC Reduces vomiting.

ANTIGALACTAGOGUE Impedes the flow of milk.

ANTIHEMORRHAGIC Helps to combat hemorrhage or bleeding.

ANTIHISTAMINE Treats allergies.

ANTI-INFECTIOUS Helps to counteract infection.

ANTI-INFLAMMATORY Prevents inflammation.

ANTILITHIC Prevents the formation of a calculus or stone.

ANTIMICROBAL Reduces microbes.

ANTINEURALGIC Reduces nerve pain.

ANTIOXIDANT Prevents or delays deterioration.

ANTIPHYLOGISTIC Reduces inflammation.

ANTIPRURITIC Prevents itching.

ANTIPUTREFACTIVE Delays the decomposition of animal and vegetable material.

ANTIPYRETIC Prevents fever.

ANTIRHEUMATIC Helps to alleviate the symptoms of rheumatism.

ANTISCLEROTIC Prevents hardening of the tissues through chronic inflammation.

ANTISCORBUTIC Helps to prevent scurvy.

ANTISEBORRHEIC Helps control the production of sebum.

ANTISEPTIC Restricts growth of bacteria.

ANTISPASMODIC Relieves smooth muscle spasms, including cramp.

ANTISUDORIFIC Counteracts perspiration.

ANTITOXIC Counteracts the effects of toxicity.

ANTITUSSIVE Relieves coughs.

ANTIVENOMOUS Counteracts poison, particularly of snakes, scorpions, or insects.

ANTIVIRAL Controls viruses.

APERITIF Stimulates appetite.

APHRODISIAC Stimulates sexual desire.

ASTRINGENT Contracts body tissues.

BACTERICIDAL Combats bacteria.

BALSAMIC Soothes and softens phlegm.

BECHIC Eases coughs.

CARDIAC Has a stimulating effect on the heart.

CARDIOTONIC Stimulates and has an affinity with the heart.

CARMINATIVE Eases griping pain and relieves flatulence.

CEPHALIC Deals with disorders of the head.

CHOLAGOGUE Stimulates the flow of bile into the duodenum.

CHOLERETIC Stimulates bile production.

CICATRISANT Promotes the formation of scar tissue.

CORDIAL A heart tonic; has an affinity with the heart.

CYTOPHYLACTIC Encourages cell regeneration.

CYTOTOXIC Poisonous to all cells.

DECONGESTANT Eases nasal mucus.

DEODORANT Prevents body odor.

DEPURATIVE Purifies the blood.

DETOXICANT Neutralizes toxic substances.

DIGESTIVE Aids digestion.

DISINFECTANT Destroys germs.

DIURETIC Stimulates the secretion of urine.

EMETIC Induces vomiting.

EMMENAGOGUE Induces or regulates menstrual flow.

EMOLLIENT Soothes and softens the skin.

ESCHAROTIC Treats warts.

EUPHORIC Induces a feeling of euphoria or well-being.

EXPECTORANT Aids the removal of catarrh.

FEBRIFUGE Reduces fever.

FIXATIVE Slows down the rate of evaporation of the more volatile ingredients of a perfume.

FUNGICIDAL Destroys fungal infections.

GALACTAGOGUE Brings on the flow of milk.

GERMICIDAL Destroys germs and micro-organisms such as bacteria.

HALLUCINOGENIC Causes visions or delusions.

HEMOSTATIC Encourages the coagulation of blood.

HEPATIC Tonic to the liver; has an affinity with the liver.

HEPATOXIC Toxic to the liver.

HYPERTENSIVE Raises the blood pressure.

HYPNOTIC Trance inducing; sleep promoting.

HYPOGLYCEMIANT Lowers blood sugar level.

HYPOTENSIVE Lowers the blood pressure.

IMMUNOSTIMULANT Stimulates the body's natural defense system.

INSECTICIDAL Kills insects.

LARVICIDAL Prevents or kills larvae.

LAXATIVE Promotes bowel evacuation.

LIPOLITIC Breaks down fat.

MUCOLYTIC Breaks down mucus.

NARCOTIC Sleep inducing; In large doses intoxicating or poisonous.

NERVINE Having a specific action on the nervous system.

NEUROTOXIC Poisonous to the nervous system.

PARASITICIDAL Discourages and eliminates parasites.

PARTURIENT Promotes and eases labor.

PEDICULICIDAL Destroys lice.

PROPHYLACTIC Helps to prevent disease.

PURGATIVE Causes evacuation of the bowels.

REGULATOR Helps to balance the functions of the body.

RELAXANT Soothes and relieves strain or tension.

RESOLVENT Dissolves boils and swellings.

RESTORATIVE Restores and revives health.

RUBEFACIENT Increases local circulation, causing the skin to redden.

SEDATIVE A nervine with a calming effect.

SIALOGOGUE Stimulates the secretion of saliva.

SOPORIFIC Induces sleep.

SPASMOLYTIC Relieves muscle cramp or spasm.

SPLENETIC A tonic to the spleen; has an affinity with the spleen.

STIMULANT Has uplifting effect on the body or mind.

STOMACHIC Relieves gastric disorders; has an affinity with the stomach.

STYPTIC Arrests external bleeding.

SUDORIFIC Induces perspiration.

TONIC Invigorates and tones the body.

UTERINE A tonic of the uterus; has an affinity with the uterus.

VASOCONSTRICTOR Local application causes contraction of the blood vessels.

VASODILATOR Local application causes dilation of the blood vessels.

VERMIFUGE Works to expel or eliminate intestinal worms.

VULNERARY Heals cuts, wounds, and sores.

Glossary of Body Systems

CARDIOVASCULAR SYSTEM

Includes the heart, the blood, the veins, the arteries, and the capillaries. As well as maintaining the flow of blood around the body, it controls the transport of oxygen from the lungs to the heart and around the organs and limbs of the body, and of carbon dioxide back to the heart and lungs.

DIGESTIVE SYSTEM

Includes the mouth, the pharynx, the esophagus, the stomach, the small and large intestines, the rectum, and the anus. It processes food from when it enters to when it leaves the body.

ENDOCRINE SYSTEM

Includes the hypothalamus, the pituitary gland, the thyroid and parathyroid glands, the pancreas, the adrenal glands, the ovaries, and the testes. The endocrine system balances hormones within the body.

LIMBIC SYSTEM

One of the earliest parts of the human brain to develop in evolutionary terms, the limbic system controls our memories, our instinct, and our vital functions. It can change objective external experience into subjective internal response.

LYMPHATIC SYSTEM

The transportation means of the immune system. Waste products carried in the lymph glands collect at lymph nodes before continuing their journey out of the body. The lymphatic system is closely connected to the cardiovascular system, but lymph, unlike blood, has no pump to drive it and so can easily become sluggish – especially in people with a particularly sedentary lifestyle.

MUSCULAR SYSTEM

This system includes every muscle of the body, plus the tendons and ligaments that link muscle to muscle and muscle to bone. It controls movement of the body.

NERVOUS SYSTEM

Includes the brain, the spinal cord, and the central nervous system. It is the system whereby physical responses to pain or sensation of any kind are transported from nerve endings in the skin to the brain. The term also includes the autonomic nervous system, which is divided into the sympathetic and

parasympathetic nervous systems. The sympathetic nervous system controls our fight/flight mechanism; it puts the body on red alert so that it can deal with danger. All the senses and responses are heightened, while the action of the digestive system slows down as it is not needed for such short-term spontaneous reactions. What happens when we submit our bodies to long-term stress is that the sympathetic nervous system is constantly activated for no reason, the result being that our body's resources are run down unnecessarily. The parasympathetic nervous system works to the opposite effect, relaxing all our stress or danger reactions and allowing the digestive system to function properly.

RESPIRATORY SYSTEM

This includes the nose, larynx, sinuses, lungs, and diaphragm. It deals with the flow of air in and out of the body.

REPRODUCTIVE SYSTEM

Includes all the male and female reproductive organs.

SKELETAL SYSTEM

The bone structure of the body.

URINARY SYSTEM

Includes the kidneys, ureters, the bladder, and the urethra. It deals with the elimination of water and waste products from the body. The reproductive system and urinary system are referred to as the genito-urinary system.

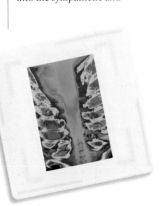

RIGHT *Different systems of the body, such as the respiratory system, respond to essential oils in different ways.*

Bibliography and Further Reading

BAERHEM, S.A. AND SCHEFFER, J.J.C, *Essential Oils and Aromatic Plants,* Dr. W. Junk Publications, 1989

DE BAIRACLI, LEVY, J., *The Illustrated Herbal Handbook,* Faber and Faber, 1982

COLVER, G. et al, *Your Skin,* Harrap, 1990

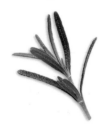

DAVIS, P., *Aromatherapy: an A to Z,* C.W. Daniel, 1991

DAVIS, P., *Subtle Aromatherapy,* C.W. Daniel, 1988

DOWNING, G., *The Massage Book,* Penguin, 1973

DYE, P., *Aromatherapy for Women and Children,* C.W. Daniel, 1992

FAWCETT, M., *Aromatherapy for Pregnancy and Childbirth,* Element, 1997

FISCHER-RIZZI, S., *Complete Aromatherapy Handbook,* Sterling, 1990

GRAYSON, J., *The Fragrant Year,* Aquarian, 1993

HOFFMAN, D., *The New Holistic Herbal,* Element Books, 1990

HOPKINS, C., *Aromatherapy,* Parallel, 1995

KAPIT, W. AND ELSON, L.M., *The Anatomy Coloring Book,* Harper Collins, 1977

LAVERY, S., *Aromatherapy in a Nutshell,* Element, 1997

LAWLESS, J., *The Complete Illustrated Guide to Aromatherapy,* Element, 1997

LAWLESS, J., *The Encyclopedia of Essential Oils,* Element, 1992

LAWLESS, J., *The Illustrated Encyclopedia of Essential Oils,* Element, 1995

LIDELL, L. et al, *The Book of Massage,* Ebury, 1984

MAXWELL-HUDSON, C., *The Complete Book of Massage,* Dorling Kindersley, 1988

MAURY, M., *Marguerite Maury's Guide to Aromatherapy,* C. W. Daniel, 1989

MOJAY, G., *Aromatherapy for Healing the Spirit,* Gaia, 1996

RICH, P., *Practical Aromatherapy,* Siena, 1996

RYMAN, D., *Aromatherapy,* Piatkus, 1991

SELLAR, W., *The Directory of Essential Oils,* C.W. Daniel, 1992

TISSERAND, R., *The Art of Aromatherapy,* C.W. Daniel, 1977

VALNET, J., *The Practice of Aromatherapy,* C.W. Daniel, 1980

WILDWOOD, C., *Encyclopedia of Essential Oils,* Bloomsbury, 1996

WORWOOD, V.A., *The Complete Book of Essential Oils,* New World Library, 1991

WORWOOD, V.A., *The Fragrant Pharmacy,* Macmillan, 1990

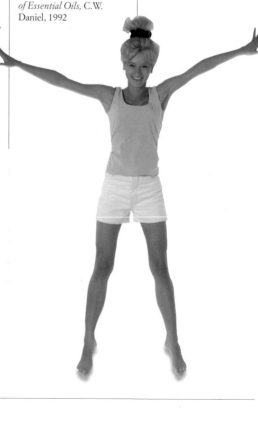

Useful Addresses

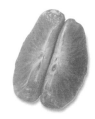

AUSTRALIA

Aromatherapy Organizations
International Federation of Aromatherapists
First Floor,
390 Burwood Road
Hawthorn
Victoria 3122

Suppliers
Essential Therapeutics
58 Easey Street
Collingwood
Victoria 3066

In Essence Aromatherapy
3 Abbott Street
Fairfield
Victoria 3078

Life Essence
70 Barbaralla Drive
Springwood
Queensland 4127

Training Courses
Margaret Tozer
Australian School of Awareness
251 Dorset Road
Croydon
Victoria 3136

CANADA

Suppliers
Green Valley Essential Oils
RR#2 Suite 205 C-6
Courtenay
British Columbia
V9N 5M9

Mother Nature's Natural Remedies
1083 Bedford Highway
Bedford
Nova Scotia
B4A 1B7

U.K.

Aromatherapy Organizations
Aromatherapy
Organisations Council
3 Latymer Close, Braybrooke
Market Harborough
Leicestershire LE16 8LN

Aromatherapy
Trades Council
P.O. Box 38
Romford
Essex RM1 2DN

International Federation
of Aromatherapists
Stamford House
2–4 Chiswick High Road
London W4 1TH

International Society
of Professional
Aromatherapists
41 Leicester Road
Hinkley LE10 1LW

Register of Qualified
Aromatherapists
P.O. Box 6941
London N8 9HF

Suppliers
Aqua Oleum
The Old Convent
Beeches Green
Stroud
Gloucestershire GL5 4AD

Baldwins
171–173 Walworth Road
London SE17 1RW

Culpepper Ltd.
34 The Pavilions
High Street
Birmingham B4 7SL

Fragrant Earth
PO Box 182
Taunton
Somerset TA1 3SD

Kittywake Oils
Cae City
Taliaris
Llandeilo
Dyfed SA19 3XA

Lothian Herbs
Peffermill Industrial Estate
Edinburgh EH16 5UY

Materia Aromatica
148 Mallinson Road
London SW11 1BJ

Neal's Yard Remedies
26–34 Ingate Place
Battersea
London SW8 3NF

Training Courses
Churchill Centre
22 Montagu Street
London W1H 1TB

Clare Maxwell Hudson Ltd.
202 Walm Lane
London NW2 3BP

Essential Care
Training Ltd.
8 George Street
Croydon
Surrey CR0 1PA

Institute of Traditional
Herbal Medicine
and Aromatherapy
PO Box 6555
London N8 9DF

London College
of Massage
5 Newman Passage
London W1P 3PF

Tisserand Institute
P.O. Box 746
Hove
Sussex BN3 3XA

Publications
Aromatherapy Quarterly
5 Ranelagh Avenue
London SW13 0BY

U.S.A.

Aromatherapy Organizations
The American Alliance of Aromatherapy
PO Box 750428
Petaluma
CA 94975

American Aromatherapy
Association
PO Box 1222
Fair Oaks
CA 95628

American Society for
Phytotherapy and
Aromatherapy
PO Box 3659
South Pasadena
CA 91031

National Association for
Holistic Aromatherapy
PO Box 17622
Boulder
CO 80308

Suppliers
Aroma Vera
3384 South
Robertson Place
Los Angeles
CA 90034

Neal's Yard U.S.A.
284 Connecticut Street
San Francisco
CA 94107

Training Courses
American Botanical Council
and Herb Research
Foundation
PO Box 201660
Austin, Texas 78720

California School of Herbal
Studies
9309 HWY116
Forestville
CA 95436

M. Das Co.
888 Brannan Street
San Francisco
CA 94103

Index